Safe and Clean Care

Infection Prevention and Control
for Health and Social Care Students

Safe and Clean Care
Infection Prevention and Control
for Health and Social Care Students

Tina Tilmouth with Simon Tilmouth

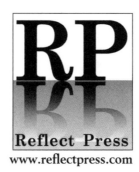

Reflect Press
www.reflectpress.com

First published in 2009

ISBN: 978 1 906052 08 9

British Library Cataloguing in Publication Data
A catalogue record for this book is available from the British Library

Production project management by Deer Park Productions

Typeset by PDQ Typesetting

Cover design by Oxmed

Printed and bound by Bell & Bain Ltd, Glasgow

Distributed by BEBC, Albion Close, Parkstone, Poole, Dorset BH12 3LL

Published by Reflect Press Ltd
11 Attwyll Avenue
Exeter
Devon, EX2 5HN
UK
01392 204400
www.reflectpress.com

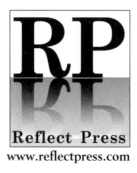

www.reflectpress.com

Contents

List of abbreviations

ACDP	Advisory Committee on Dangerous Pathogens
AIDS	Acquired Immune Deficiency Syndrome
APIC	Association for Professionals in Infection Control and Epidemiology (USA)
AZT	azidothymidine
BSE	bovine spongiform encephalitis
BSI	body substance isolation
CCDC	Consultant in Communicable Disease Control
CDC	Centers for Disease Control and Prevention (USA)
CDSC	Communicable Disease Surveillance Centre (Northern Ireland)
CHAI	Commission for Health Care Audit and Inspection
CHI	Commission for Health Improvement
CICN	community infection control nurse
CJD	Creutzfeldt-Jacob disease
COSHH	Control of Substances Hazardous to Health Regulations 2002
CSCI	Commission for Social Care Inspection
DHQP	Division of Healthcare Quality Promotion (USA)
DNA	deoxyribonucleic acid – the genetic material of all living organisms
DoH	Department of Health
EHPs	environmental health practitioners
EPIC	evidence-based practice in infection control
EPO	Environmental Protection Office
ESBLs	extended-spectrum ß lactamases
GRE	glycopeptide-resistant enterococci
HBV	hepatitis B virus

HCAI/HAI	health-care associated infection
HCC	Health Care Commission
HIS	Hospital Infection Society
HIV	human immunodeficiency virus
HPA	Health Protection Agency
HSE	Health and Safety Executive
ICC	infection control committee
ICD	infection control doctor
ICN	infection control nurse
ICNA	Infection Control Nurses Association
ICT	infection control team
IPS	Infection Prevention Society
MDA	Medical Devices Agency
MDR-TB	multidrug-resistant tuberculosis
MMR	mumps, measles and rubella [vaccine]
MRSA	methicillin-resistant *Staphylococcus aureus*
NHS	National Health Service
NICE	National Institute for Health and Clinical Excellence
NMC	Nursing and Midwifery Council
NPHS	National Public Health Service (Wales)
NSO	National Statistics Office (now the ONS)
ONS	Office for National Statistics
PCT	Primary Care Trust
PPE	personal protective equipment
RCN	Royal College of Nursing
RIDDOR	Reporting of Injuries, Diseases and Dangerous Occurrences Regulations 1995
RNA	ribonucleic acid
SARS	severe acute respiratory syndrome
SHTAC	Scottish Health and Technology Assessment Centre
SpHA	special health authority
TB	tuberculosis
VRE	vancomycin-resistant enterococci
WHO	World Health Organization
XDR-TB	extensively drug-resistant tuberculosis

Introduction

Despite all the advances in modern care and medical technology the simple fact remains: people still die from infective disorders that can be prevented by standard measures. The Chief Medical Officer's report *Winning Ways: Working Together to Reduce Healthcare Associated Infection in England* (DoH, 2003c) estimates that 15 to 20 per cent of HCAI (health-care associated infection) is preventable.

The increase in the number of HCAIs and the rise in the cost of treating these have led to a number of initiatives proposed by government and health care professionals. New legislation and changed priorities for care settings have inevitably led to the need to alter the way in which care workers are trained and the way in which they work.

REFERENCING THE STANDARDS

This book, specifically prepared for health and social care workers in various settings, has used the Skills for Care Knowledge Set for Infection Prevention and Control, the Skills for Health Infection Prevention and Control Competencies and the Essential Skills Clusters prepared by the Nursing and Midwifery Council (NMC) as the basis for the key learning outcomes in this resource. The Skills for Care Knowledge Sets provide key learning outcomes for specific areas of work within the adult care sector. The knowledge sets have been designed to improve the consistency in care in the adult social care sector and there are similar initiatives for other care workers in health care settings. The Skills for Health competencies, the Essential Skills Clusters produced by the NMC and the EPIC project (evidence-based practice in infection control), are guidelines that have been developed to address the problems we encounter with infection control in health care environments.

CONTENT AND COVERAGE

The outcomes provide the minimum standards employers need to reach when either designing or using other training resources. This book with its format of exercises, case studies and reflective activities will provide the opportunity for staff working through it to build up a portfolio of evidence to meet the knowledge set and competency standards. Each chapter highlights the outcomes to be covered and provides exercises that can be used to test the achievement of these outcomes.

Designed specifically for people who work in the health and social care sector this textbook will also prove very useful for those undertaking a Foundation Degree in Health and Social Care. For teachers of A Level and Foundation Degree Health courses, the book will provide up-to-date materials which deal with the new initiatives in controlling and preventing infection. The activities can be used in classroom settings and answers are provided at the end of each chapter.

Chapter 1

In Chapter 1 the reader is introduced to the microbiological aspects of infection and will consider how infection is spread through the chain of infection. The content will cover the definition of infection and colonisation, the difference between pathogens and parasites and the growth of such micro-organisms. Its accessible style will enable the reader to understand the more complex areas of microbiology by applying them to the practice they undertake on a daily basis. The author of this chapter is the Head of Biology at a large 'Beacon' Sixth Form College and has a wealth of experience teaching A Level Biology and Human Biology in addition to working for a major examining board. His style of writing and the application to the care setting brings the subject alive and demonstrates the practicalities of the links between microbiology and the workplace.

Chapter 2

Chapter 2 demonstrates how the problems associated with HCAIs affect our society today. Communicable disease such as tuberculosis (TB), influenza and legionnaires' disease are also addressed and the rates of infection in hospitals and the community are covered, together with identifying who is at risk and why. The effects of infection on patients and clients will also be highlighted. This chapter deals with the state of our care settings at this moment in time and tries to point out how we have arrived at this level of infection. With just a brief look at the historical view the reader will find the chapter invaluable in sourcing some of the government initiatives that are designed to deal with the current problem.

Chapter 3

Chapter 3 deals primarily with the legislation, regulations and guidance that we as care workers need to access in order to address the rise in infection. A variety of laws and initiatives and the key standards and guidance are covered in this chapter. We will address the ways in which clinical governance has impacted upon the care setting and look in some detail at the various policies we work with and how they can help to shape our understanding of the way in which we practice.

Standard precautions, risk assessment and the EPIC guidelines are all introduced in this chapter and the activities will ensure that you have access to the relevant documents you may require in your work setting.

Chapter 4

Cleaning and waste management has seen a change in recent years and is a major area where infection can be transmitted. Chapter 4 sets out to show the standard precautions to prevent infection and its spread as well as the correct procedures for the handling, storage and disposal of waste (using the correct colour-coded bag or bin and decontamination techniques). The importance of hand hygiene as one of the most effective ways of ensuring that cross infection is minimised and the use of protective equipment, not only for the patient/client but also for the care worker, is clearly outlined.

The Code of Practice for the Prevention and Control of Healthcare Associated Infections ensures that NHS bodies have a duty to provide and maintain a clean and appropriate environment and the Deep Clean Initiative is just one of a wide range of measures introduced by the government that will be covered in this chapter. Also, with respect to the generation of waste in terms of towels, dressings, needles and syringes as well as linen and bodily waste, the chapter will introduce you to the Controlled Waste Regulations 1992, which give us guidance as to how to ensure we follow correct procedures in this.

Chapter 5

Chapter 5 looks at the government guidance and legislation that deals with keeping yourself and your service users safe in the working environment. The need for safety policies and risk assessment under the requirements of Health and Safety at Work Regulations 1999 (Management Regulation) is also addressed here. The Reporting of Injuries Disease and Dangerous Occurrence Regulations 1995 (RIDDOR) guidance and the Control of Substances Hazardous to Health Regulations 2002 (COSHH) regulations are discussed and the need for accurate record-keeping is emphasised.

Chapter 6

In the final chapter the responsibilities and roles in infection control are discussed. Many changes in the NHS in 2000 saw the services being moved from the District Health Authority to newly formed Primary Care Trusts. Strategic Health Authorities replaced the old regional health authorities and Public Health Leadership became firmly the role of the Directors for Public Health. At Trust level the chief executive ensures that there are arrangements in place for the control of infection in the Trust and that programmes are implemented and monitored by specialist staff. In the social care setting the roles and responsibilities are identified in the Department of Health document entitled *Infection Control Guidance for Care Homes* (DoH, 2006a). In line with the require-ments set out by the Health Act 2006, the responsibilities with respect to all aspects of infection control are clearly identified and in this chapter you will learn who is responsible in your setting for the arrangements for safe working with respect to infection control.

AUTHOR BIOGRAPHIES

Tina Tilmouth

Tina, a Registered General Nurse and experienced teacher, currently holds the post of Programme Leader for Health and Social Care at Ludlow Sixth Form College. She has authored several distance learning texts including those for NVQ Level Two, Three, the Registered Managers Award and the Safe Handling of Medicines. Previously she wrote a text for the Open College Network about the use of Contract Learning in Nurse Education (1989). Tina teaches on a range of health care subjects for students from 14 years to 19+ and has links with Worcester University through the Foundation Degree in Health and Social Care.

Simon Tilmouth

Simon is the current Head of Biology at Shrewsbury Sixth Form College and also works for a major examining board.

Chapter 1

What is Infection: How is it Spread, Controlled and Prevented?

In this chapter you will cover the following standards and competencies:

- Skills for Care Knowledge Set on Infection Prevention and Control
  1. Cause and spread of infection
     - 1.1 Understand the definition of infection and colonisation
     - 1.2 Understand how micro-organisms cause infection
     - 1.3 Understand the essential differences between pathogenic micro-organisms and parasitic organisms, and the diseases they cause
     - 1.4 Understand how pathogenic micro-organisms grow and spread.
- Skills for Health Infection Prevention and Control Competencies: IPC1
  Knowledge and understanding
  K4 A factual knowledge of the chain of infection.

INTRODUCTION

A woman has become the first nurse in England to be struck off for failing to wash her hands after treating a patient with MRSA.
(http://news.bbc.co.uk/1/hi/england/7108925.stm)

Case Study 1

Typhoid Mary

How would you feel if a stranger approached you and asked for samples of your blood, faeces and urine? This was the situation faced by Mary Mallon in March 1907 when George Soper confronted her at her place of work.

Soper had been hired by George Thompson to investigate the cause of an outbreak of typhoid fever at his summer home in Long Island, New

York. Soper suspected that Mallon, hired as a cook at the summer home, was the cause of infection and had traced her employment history back to 1900. He found that typhoid outbreaks had followed Mary from job to job and that in seven jobs 22 people had become ill and one young girl had died.

In order to confirm his suspicions Soper needed to analyse blood and stool samples for the presence of *Salmonella typhi*, the bacterium that causes typhoid fever.

Eventually, after several encounters and the support of five police officers, Mallon was taken into the Willard Parker Hospital in New York and a stool sample obtained. *Salmonella typhi* was found in the sample and Mallon was, against her will, transferred to an isolated cottage on North Brother Island, New York. She remained there for two years and, during this time, 120 of 163 stool samples taken tested positive for the pathogen.

In February 1910 Mary was released with the condition that she never worked as a cook again.

In January 1915 the Sloane Maternity Hospital in Manhattan suffered a typhoid outbreak. Twenty-five people became ill and two of them died. Evidence pointed to a recently hired cook Mrs Brown. Mrs Brown turned out to be Mary Mallon working under an assumed name. Mary was again sent to North Brother Island where she remained until her death (not of typhoid fever) in 1938.

(http://history1900s.about.com/od/1900s/a/typhoidmary.htm)

Apart from the ethical issues of imprisoning a woman who initially had not broken the law what does this case study illustrate?

- The need for rigorous hygiene – especially when dealing with food – as disease can be spread via unwashed hands.
- People can be carriers of a disease without suffering from that disease. Mallon was not infected but she was colonised. There is a clear and important distinction between infection and colonisation. The people that became ill from the bacteria that Mallon transmitted to them were clearly infected. So the difference is that infected people have the bacteria and get sick and colonised people have the bacteria and don't. There is more on this later in the chapter.

When we think of disease we often think of something we can catch and therefore assume that disease is infectious. As health care professionals you will of course be aware of other disease types and their causes. Cystic fibrosis is inherited, osteoporosis is a degenerative disease and cancer has inherited, degenerative and environmental influences. This chapter is going to consider infectious diseases, the micro-organisms or pathogens that cause them, other factors that may contribute to the incidence of the disease and the ways in which the pathogens are spread. As with the typhoid fever example, case studies will be used to illustrate some of the aspects of infectious disease.

CELL BIOLOGY (CYTOLOGY)

In order to understand how diseases are caused, together with their signs and symptoms, we should first consider some basic cell biology or **cytology**. The cell theory states that all living things are cellular, be they unicellular like bacteria or multicellular like humans (viruses do not have a cellular structure and as such are not classified as living).

A human body consists of somewhere in the region of 50 trillion cells. So what does that really mean? A trillion is a thousand billion, which is a thousand million. If cells were pounds and you were to spend ten thousand pounds a day every day it would take you nearly 14 million years to spend it all and that's without any accumulated interest! Yet it is estimated that there are in fact more bacterial cells in and on you than there are human cells. These cells are rather simple in structure when compared with human cells yet they are incredibly numerous, incredibly small (around 1/1000 of a millimetre) and can be lethal. It has been estimated that 1 ml of culture fluid of *Clostridium botulinum* is sufficient to kill two million mice and that the lethal dose for humans may be around 1 µg of botulinum toxin – that is one thousandth of a gram (Volk *et al.*, 1991).

Not all bacteria cause disease and those that do often need very specific conditions to thrive and become **pathogenic** (disease-causing). In fact, many bacteria are positively beneficial to us. For example, our large intestines harbour a large population of *Escherichia coli* producing vitamin K that we absorb and use.

The numbers of bacteria and other microbes, their relative invisibility and their rapid reproduction rate make the task of controlling them very difficult indeed. However, if we understand how they work, the conditions they require to thrive and reproduce and how they are transmitted we can go a long way towards controlling the diseases they cause.

Bacteria have a particular cell type and are termed the **prokaryotes**. All bacteria are prokaryotes and all prokaryotes are bacteria so therefore, throughout this chapter, bacteria/bacterium will be used to refer to prokaryotic organisms. All other living organisms have a more complex cell type and are termed **eukaryotes**.

Prokaryotes

Prokaryotes are unicellular – that is, one bacterium consists of one cell. However, they do form colonies or groupings that can be used in their classification and subsequent identification. The size of an average bacterium is 1 micrometre (µm) or a thousandth of a millimetre. They are incredibly numerous (it has been estimated that a gram of soil contains one hundred million living bacteria (Postgate, 1992)) and reproduce very rapidly – some have a generation time of 20 minutes and, if left to reproduce without limits, would produce a colony in three days that weighs more that the planet (Postgate, 1992). Fortunately, something will always limit their growth and reproduction rate and prevent the rather terrifying prospect of us being overrun by a mass of bacteria. However, their rate of growth can be truly extraordinary.

Activity 1

If you start with one bacterium that reproduces every 20 minutes, how many bacteria would you have after eight hours? So, after 20 minutes you would have two, after 40 minutes you would have four and so on.

(Answers to all relevant Activities are given at the end of the chapter.)

The horizontal transfer of genes

One significant characteristic of bacteria is the horizontal transfer of genes. As humans we transfer our genes and characteristics to our children via sexual reproduction. Our genes are present in our sperm and eggs and combine at fertilisation to produce a cell that develops into a new person. The genes present in the sperm and egg largely control the characteristics of this person. Bacteria can also transfer their genes and subsequent characteristics from individual to individual. However, a gene for antibiotic resistance can be spread throughout an existing population of bacteria without the need for sexual reproduction. This is akin to you transferring the gene you possess for blue/brown/grey/green eyes to your friend or partner who then assumes that characteristic. The horizontal transfer of genes will be covered in more detail later in this chapter.

Commensal bacteria

One more thing to consider before we look at the detailed structure of a typical bacterium is that not all bacteria are bad. Some bacteria are good and live in and on us to our mutual benefit. These are referred to as **commensal** bacteria and, while they may consume some of our food if they live in our intestine, they may also help to keep any pathogenic bacteria in check.

The cell structure of prokaryotes

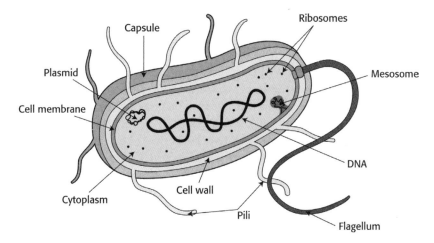

Figure 1 A bacterium

Figure 1 is a diagram showing the basic structure of a bacterium cell. All living organisms share some characteristics such as movement, a way of gaining nutrients and the ability to break them down to release the energy contained in them. Clearly different species of organism have different characteristics such as feathers in birds, the eight legs of an octopus, etc. Equally obvious is the variation present when considering a characteristic within any particular species. These characteristics and varieties are controlled by **genes**. Genes are lengths of DNA that tell the cell how to make a particular protein. This protein then controls the characteristics and functioning of the organism. For example, in human saliva there is a protein that breaks down starch present in our food – it is called amylase and belongs to a group of proteins called **enzymes** that are involved in the majority of chemical reactions that occur in living organisms. So the ability to digest starch is determined by the presence of a particular gene that contains the genetic code for the enzyme amylase. Other genes code for the ability to roll your tongue, the colour of your eyes, your blood group, etc. Other proteins may be involved in movement like, for example, muscle protein or act as hormones such as, for example, insulin.

Proteins are made within the cell using a complicated set of machinery that differs between human cells and bacterial cells. These differences are important when we come to consider the use of antibiotics and how they kill bacterial cells but not human cells. The biological machinery within a bacterium is as follows.

Cell wall

The cell wall stops the bacterium from bursting. Water will move into the cell by a process called osmosis. This is because the concentration of water within the bacterium is often lower than that in the environment. The cell wall is there to stop the cell popping like a balloon. There are variations in the structure of bacterial cells walls – these variations are useful in laboratory identification where they will stain different colours. For example, some bacteria have a very thick cell wall and stain violet when using a technique called **Gram staining** – these are referred to as **Gram positive** bacteria. Other bacteria have a thinner wall but have an extra layer of lipids on the outside. These stain pink when using the Gram staining technique and are referred to as **Gram negative** bacteria. The significance of this particular technique is that Gram positive and Gram negative bacteria respond to different groups of antibiotics so this technique can ensure the correct antibiotic is prescribed for a particular infection.

The cell membrane

The cell membrane regulates what enters and leaves the cell. Certain molecules within the membrane act as **antigens**. These molecules are recognised by our immune system and stimulate an immune response.

Mesosome

The mesosome is a folding of the membrane and is the site of respiration in the cell, i.e. where food is broken down to release energy.

DNA

DNA – deoxyribose nucleic acid – is the very stuff of life. This molecule contains the instructions on how to make proteins. As mentioned above, these proteins control the characteristics of the bacterium.

Ribosomes

Ribosomes are the protein-making machines. Human cells have them as well although they differ in size.

Cytoplasm

Cytoplasm is a solution of chemicals such as simple sugars and amino acids and a suspension of larger organic molecules.

Flagella

Flagella are used for locomotion.

Plasmids

Plasmids are small loops of DNA that can be transferred to other bacteria. The transfer of plasmids from bacterium to bacterium is the horizontal transfer of genes mentioned above.

Eukaryotes

The eukaryotes include all other living organisms – humans and all other animals, plants, fungi, seaweeds, etc. Eukaryotic cells have a more complex structure than that of prokaryotic cells, with some significant differences that can be used to distinguish between host cells and prokaryotic cells in the treatment of bacterial infections.

The structure of a typical eukaryotic cell

Figure 2 depicts the structure of a typical eukaryotic cell.

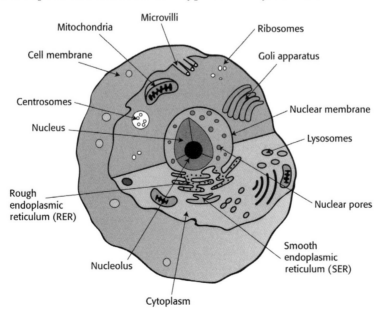

Figure 2 The structure of a typical human eukaryotic cell

Cell membrane

The cell membrane regulates what enters and leaves the cell.

Microvilli

Microvilli are folds in the membrane that increase the surface area of the cell for absorption. For example, the cells lining the human gut have microvilli for the absorption of water and the products of digestion.

Mitochondrion

The mitochondria are the site of respiration, i.e. where simple organic molecules are broken down to release energy.

Lysosome

A lysosome is a bag made from cell membrane. It contains digestive enzymes and is used in phagocytes to kill and digest bacteria (see below).

Rough endoplasmic reticulum

The rough endoplasmic reticulum is a network of membranes that has ribosomes on the surface. Ribosomes make proteins.

Smooth endoplasmic reticulum

The smooth endoplasmic reticulum is a network of membranes without ribosomes. This is the site of steroid synthesis – for example, testosterone.

Golgi apparatus

The Golgi apparatus is the dispatch department. Anything to be secreted from the cell comes through here – for example, insulin secreted into the blood.

Nucleus

By definition all eukaryotes have nuclei in their cells. Chromosomes within the nucleus contain DNA/genes.

In summary, all living organisms, be they human or bacteria, are cellular. The detailed structure of the cells enables these organisms to survive and reproduce. The differences between the prokaryotes and eukaryotes can be used as targets when treating bacterial infections (see antibiotics below).

VIRUSES

Viruses are not considered to be living organisms. One key fact is that they cannot reproduce on their own – they lack the complex ultrastructure of prokaryotes and eukaryotes. Viruses consist of a nucleic acid (DNA or a similar molecule called RNA) that contains the viral genes and a protein coat or capsid (see Figure 3).

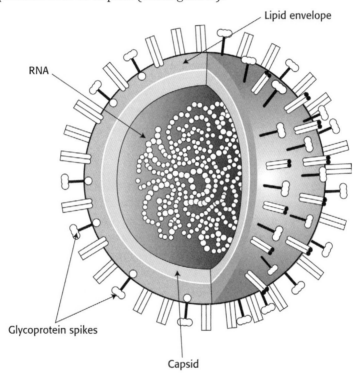

Figure 3 The influenza virus

In addition, some viruses may have another lipid envelope. They lack any of the machinery to translate the information contained in their genes into functional proteins.

So how do they reproduce and make us ill? Quite simply, they enter the cell and take over (see Figure 4). They order the cell to make new viruses and viral proteins using the energy, raw materials and machinery of the cell. The cell becomes a factory for making viral proteins and new viruses. These are then released ready to infect another cell and this may cause the destruction of the cell.

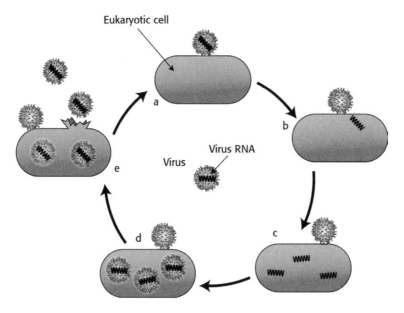

Figure 4 Viral reproduction

Let's consider influenza as a viral disease to illustrate the viral cycle of infection. There are three types of influenza virus A, B and C. These viruses have RNA as their genetic material and have a lipid coat or envelope with spikes that enable them to attach to and penetrate the host's respiratory mucous membranes. They replicate here and cause the normal symptoms of flu – fever, cough, aches and pains, etc. Secondary bacterial infections resulting from a viral infection can often be more serious and can lead to death.

THE REPRODUCTION OF BACTERIA AND VIRUSES

As described above, viruses hijack the protein-making machinery of other cells in order to replicate. The viral particles can then be spread via the normal routes such as, for example, direct contact, airborne droplets or the oral/faecal route.

Bacterial reproduction is termed binary fission – this literally means splitting in two. The bacterium copies its DNA and then splits into two cells, each with the correct amount of DNA. Human cells replicate in a similar way when tissues grow or repair. This process may be preceded or not by the horizontal transfer of genes as described on page 4.

Bacteria can also produce **endospores**. These are produced within the bacterium and are released into the environment where they can remain dormant for thousands of years. They are more resistant to fluctuations in environmental conditions such as extremes of temperature, lack of water, etc. For example, most bacteria are killed by temperatures above 70°C but spores can survive in boiling water for several hours. These spores can then germinate when conditions are suitable and become active bacteria.

PATHOGENICITY, ROUTES OF TRANSMISSION AND IMMUNOLOGY

Infection and colonisation

Before we go any further we need to define some terms with respect to microbes and disease. We must distinguish between infection and colonisation. We all harbour a vast number of different micro-organisms that inhabit our digestive tract, the surface of our skin and parts of our reproductive system. These micro-organisms are termed our normal 'flora'; they do us little harm and, in fact, many are positively beneficial to our health. For example, the vagina contains large numbers of bacteria that produce lactic acid. This restricts the growth of other pathogenic organisms such as *Candida albicans* (the fungus that causes thrush). Some gut bacteria produce essential vitamins or indeed help to break down our food. These are examples of commensal bacteria as they provide a benefit to us as the host. Therefore we are all colonised by bacteria.

Pathogenicity

However, our main concern in this book is those bacteria, fungi and viruses that cause infection/disease – these are termed **pathogens**. What sets apart pathogens from other micro-organisms and what properties do they have that make them pathogenic?

While some infectious diseases are caused by a bite or a wound, many infections are spread via the mucous membranes – that is the lining of body cavities that open to the outside. This includes the respiratory, digestive and reproductive tracts. The first requirement then is for bacteria to *survive* on mucous membranes. In some cases survival here may be enough to cause disease but many bacteria will need to *penetrate* the mucous membrane in order to gain entry to the body and infect us.

Once inside the host pathogens must be able to *reproduce* in order to become pathogenic. The internal environment of a human being is a wonderful place for pathogens in as much as that the environment is temperature controlled and has a constant supply of nutrients and water. However, potential pathogens also have to be able to *resist* the defences of the host. These defences are numerous and include inflammation, pathogen-eating cells called **phagocytes** and proteins such as **complement** and antibodies that destroy pathogens. The ability to *damage* the host is the final act in the repertoire of the pathogen. This can be achieved by the production of bacterial toxins that cause, for example, the vomiting and diarrhoea in cholera.

The cholera pathogen *Vibrio cholerae* secretes a toxin that blocks the absorption of food and water from the intestine. This results in diarrhoea and vomiting that can be lethal for the person infected and that transmits the bacterium to another host. The HIV virus destroys cells during the act of viral replication. As discussed above, viruses take over cells and use the cells' ultrastructure to make new viruses. The release of these newly formed viruses may result in the destruction of that cell. In the case of HIV and AIDS the cells that are host to the HIV are a crucial part of the immune system (they are known as CD4 helper cells). The HIV virus targets these particular cells by having a protein in its lipid envelope that fits with a protein on the surface of these particular CD4 helper cells – they fit like a lock and key. When this happens the virus is taken into the cell. The destruction of the CD4 helper cells compromises immune function and secondary infections and tumours can develop, leading to AIDS. Pathogens can also cause disease by stimulating an immune response that actually does more harm than good like, for example, in the tubercles of TB (Smith, 1995).

Activity 2

The use of mnemonics as memory tools can be very useful. 'Richard Of York Gave Battle in Vain' is a classic example of a mnemonic that helps school children remember the colours of the rainbow in the correct order.

Construct your own mnemonic to help you to remember the five requirements of pathogenicity given in italics in the text above.

Routes of transmission

Infectious disease, by definition, can be transmitted from one person to another. There are four main ways in which this can happen and these are known as the routes of transmission.

The oral/faecal route

The pathogen or its **spores** are present in the faeces of a carrier or sufferer in incredible numbers. For example, a person with cholera excretes 10 000 000 000 000 bacteria every day in faeces and vomit. The number of bacteria required to cause the disease in someone else is around 1 000 000 (a million). This sounds a lot – and it is – yet one person could, in theory, infect 10 million other people every day (Jones, 1994). Typhoid Mary (see Case study 1) is an example of a carrier who was transmitting the disease via this particular route. Bacteria in her faeces were transmitted to the food she served and, subsequently, to the people who ate it. In Chapter 3 we will look more closely at how hand washing is a major factor in preventing cross infection. As a cook Mary Mallon was obviously not aware of this. However, the nurse who was the subject of the headline at the beginning of this chapter surely was!

The airborne route by droplet infection

The pathogen or its spores are present in the air and are inhaled by another person. These may well have just left the carrier/sufferer via a cough or sneeze or spores may be present in the environment like, for example, in bedding. Tuberculosis is a good example of a pathogen that is mainly spread this way.

Direct contact

This method covers a range of possibilities. The transmission of syphilis or chlamydia via unprotected sexual intercourse is an example as is the transmission of HIV by sharing needles.

Via a vector

In this sense a vector is an organism that transmits the pathogen to a person via a bite. For example, malaria is caused by a unicellular eukaryotic organism of the genus *Plasmodium*. This pathogen is transmitted from one person to another by a female mosquito of the genus *Anopheles* that is acting as the vector.

Some diseases can be transmitted via more than one route; for example, TB can be spread via droplet inhalation and is occasionally spread via direct contact.

As we have established, bacteria and viruses are everywhere and we come into contact with them every day. Why are we generally so healthy and not constantly suffering from bacterial or viral infections? We have established that not all micro-organisms are pathogenic but, to fully answer this question, we need to consider some basic aspects of the human immune system.

A brief guide to immunity

The immune system can be regarded as having three lines of defence (see Figure 5):

1. physical/chemical barriers to prevent infection;
2. the non-specific immune response – targeted at anything that shouldn't be in the body;
3. the specific immune response – targeted at a specific pathogen.

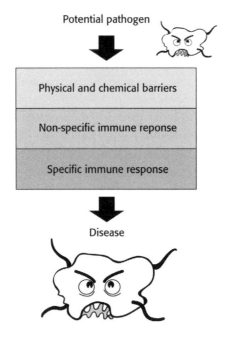

Figure 5 The human immune system

Physical/chemical barriers to infection

In many ways the internal environment of our bodies provides an ideal habitat for pathogens. It is warm, wet and has a constant supply of nutrients. To gain entry to this constant, nutrient-rich environment pathogens must first overcome a range of both physical and chemical barriers. The first and largest barrier to infection is the skin – this provides a relatively tough and impermeable barrier to infection. The outermost layer of the skin – the epidermis – produces a protein called keratin that is largely responsible for this barrier-like quality. Secretions such as sebum from the sebaceous glands also inhibit the growth of certain bacteria.

However, the skin has openings that all offer an opportunity for bacteria and other pathogens to gain access. These openings have their own barriers to infection and a brief outline of each follows.

The digestive tract

Within saliva there is an antibacterial enzyme called lysozyme that breaks down the cell wall of some bacteria. In addition, gastric juice found in the stomach has a pH of 1.5 (very acidic) – this kills the majority of pathogens that are ingested.

The eyes

Tears also contain the enzyme lysozyme.

The ears

Earwax or cerumen is antibacterial.

The respiratory tract

All body cavities that open directly to the exterior are lined with mucous membranes. Therefore the digestive, respiratory, reproductive and urinary tracts are lined with mucous membranes. These membranes have common features and also some unique properties depending on their location. For example, the secretion of mucous in the digestive tract lubricates the passage of food but, in the respiratory tract, mucous membranes trap dirt and possible pathogens. This mucous is wafted up the respiratory tract by hair-like structures called cilia that beat in unison and are found in the cells making up the mucous membrane. The mucous is moved in this way to the mouth where it can then be swallowed and the stomach acid takes care of the pathogens.

The reproductive/urinary tract

The vagina has a low pH that acts as a barrier to infection. Also, the flow of urine in both males and females inhibits urinary tract infections.

As we are all too aware these barriers don't always work! As we have already seen, the oral/faecal route can spread pathogens – so some pathogens are clearly unaffected by stomach acid. Similarly, the mucous membranes are not always effective against pathogens that are airborne. Direct contact may result in the mucous membrane being breached via a cut or a vector may penetrate the skin allowing the pathogen to gain entry.

When inside the human body the pathogen then has to survive a whole range of physiological responses that may be targeted at anything that shouldn't be there (non-specific response) or may in fact be targeted very specifically at a particular pathogen (specific response). The question is, how does the body know that these pathogens shouldn't be there?

The non-specific immune response

On the surface of every cell, be it pathogen or human, are protein molecules that identify the cell as 'self' or 'non-self' to our immune system. Our cells have these molecules, called **antigens**, which tell our immune system 'this is part of us ("self") so leave alone'. However, pathogens have differently shaped antigens that tell the immune system 'this is not part of us ("non-self") so attack'.

The first non-specific response is by white blood cells called phagocytes (see Figure 6). These cells engulf and digest any pathogen that they come across. Other non-specific immune responses include fever and inflammation. Fever inhibits the growth of bacteria by increasing the temperature to a level that inhibits the pathogen's physiology. Inflammation increases blood flow to the infected area, thereby increasing the supply of both phagocytes and non-specific antibacterial proteins such as complement. Complement is a set of proteins that bind to pathogens/antigens and promote phagocytosis.

The specific immune response

The specific immune response is also dependent on the antigens on the surface of pathogens being recognised by the body. A group of white blood cells called lymphocytes are largely responsible for the specific immune response. They reside in lymph tissue and are activated by the presence of a specific pathogen antigen. This sets in motion a complex series of chemical reactions and cell divisions. Ultimately what are produced are antibodies and killer cells. Antibodies are protein molecules produced by B lymphocytes. They fit the antigen like a lock fits a key – that is they are specific to only one type or shape of antigen. They are released into the blood stream by the million and move within the circulatory system binding to the specific antigen whenever it is encountered.

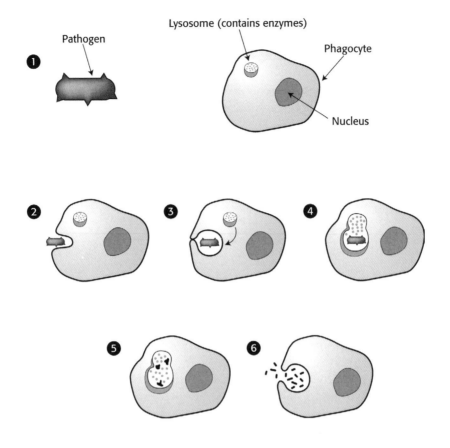

Figure 6 The action of phagocytes

Antibodies may cause the breakdown or clumping (agglutination) of bacteria. When agglutination has occurred they are then destroyed by phagocytes. Antibodies can also neutralise any toxins produced.

Another type of lymphocyte, the T lymphocyte, is activated by the presence of specific antigens and produces killer T cells. These cells specifically bind to and destroy the pathogen.

When B and T lymphocytes are activated not only are antibodies and killer T cells produced but also memory B cells and memory T cells. These are responsible for long-term immunity and remain in your lymph system indefinitely. When the same pathogen (with the same antigen) is encountered again they respond very quickly and very vigorously. This deals with the infection before signs and symptoms develop (see Figure 7).

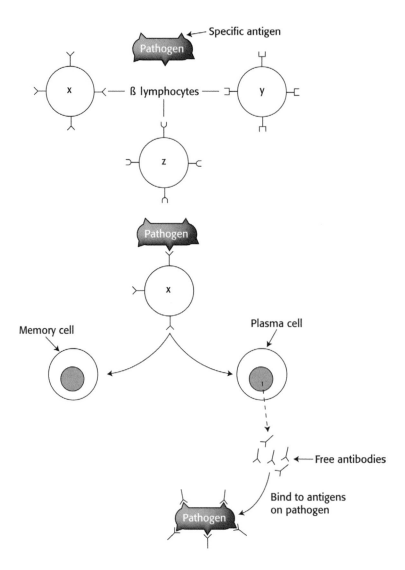

Figure 7 The action of lymphocytes

Through natural mutation the pathogens' antigens may change shape and therefore manage to avoid the memory cells produced when this pathogen was originally detected. When this happens, as with the case of influenza, the immune system has to go through the whole recognition process again.

The purpose of vaccination is to stimulate the production of memory cells without giving you the disease.

Activity 3

A vaccine may give long-term or active immunity. There are three types of vaccine that vary in their contents. Research the three types and the ways in which they stimulate the production of memory cells.

BACTERIAL NAMES

Why do bacteria have such long names? The 'long names' are not confined to bacteria but apply to all living organisms. For example, humans are *Homo sapiens*. *Homo* is the genus – a grouping that may include several species such as *sapiens*. In the case of the genus *Homo* the species *sapiens* is the only surviving species. The bacterium that causes tetanus is *Clostridium tetani* – genus *Clostridium*, species *tetani*. There are other species of this genus such as, for example, *Clostridium difficile* – genus *Clostridium*, species *difficile*. Organisms that have the same genus are more closely related and share more characteristics than organisms that do not.

Therefore, all living organisms have a scientific name consisting of two words – this is known as the **binomen** or **binary combination** and should be either italicised or underlined when written with the genus having a capital letter. This system of naming is international and independent of the language spoken in any country therefore *Escherichia coli* in Sweden refers to the same bacterium as *Escherichia coli* in Japan.

Case Study 2

Clostridium difficile

Clostridium difficile (C. *difficile* or C. *diff*) is a major cause of diarrhoea and colitis (bleeding from the colon), mainly in elderly patients with other diseases that have been treated with broad spectrum antibiotics.

This bacterium is an **anaerobe**, which means that it can only survive in environments without oxygen. However, it produces **spores** that can survive for a long time in the environment and can result in the transmission of the disease. It can be present at low levels in the intestine of healthy people of all ages where competition with the other bacteria present keeps the population in check at a non-pathogenic level. If these other bacteria are killed by the use of a broad spectrum antibiotic to treat another disease then the C. *difficile* bacteria multiply to pathogenic levels. The bacterium produces two toxins that damage the cells lining the intestine, causing diarrhoea that can range from a mild case to ulceration, colitis and even peritonitis resulting from the perforation of the intestine. The diarrhoea of infected patients contains large numbers of C. *difficile* spores that can contaminate the environment and can result in the spread of the disease.

The incidence of C. *difficile* infections has increased rapidly since the early 1990s and it is now part of the mandatory surveillance programme for health care associated infections. A mutated form of the bacterium has evolved that produces greater amounts of toxin than the original form. This is type 027 and produces more severe cases and a higher mortality rate. The Department of Health recommends three main steps in the control of C. *difficile* infections.

1. A reduction in the prescription of broad spectrum antibiotics.

2. Isolation of patients with C. *difficile* diarrhoea and good infection control.

3. Enhanced environmental cleaning.

(DoH, 2007a)

Case Study 3

Tuberculosis

More than 70 per cent of Europeans were infected with TB at one time or other during the 1800s. Approximately one in seven died of the disease and many of these people were immigrants, industrial workers or the homeless. In fact, with the exception of AIDS patients, the same sort of people die of TB today (Nikiforuk, 1991).

Worldwide TB is a massive problem. In England the incidence of TB was in decline until the mid-1980s but started to rise again in the early 1990s. In 2006, there were 8497 reported cases of TB in the UK (14 per 100 000) with the London region accounting for 40 per cent of cases (**www.dh.gov.uk/en/Publichealth/Communicablediseases/Tuberculosis/index.htm**).

The Department of Health attribute the decline of TB to 'better nutrition and housing; pasteurisation of milk; the introduction of effective drug treatments; early detection through mass miniature X-ray programmes; public health programmes to detect and treat infection in close contacts of people with newly diagnosed TB; and BCG immunisation' (DoH, 2004d). The increase in TB from the early 1990s is attributed to an increase in immigration from areas of the world where TB is more prevalent. Aging of the existing population and the incidence of TB in HIV positive people also make small but important contributions to the overall total (DoH, 2004d).

All forms of TB are compulsorily notifiable under the Public Health (Control of Disease) Act 1984.

WHAT IS TB?

TB, tuberculosis, the white plague and consumption are all names for the disease that is caused by bacteria of the genus *Mycobacterium*. *M. tuberculosis* is the main cause of the disease in humans – it is an **aerobe** (needs oxygen) and is spread via inhaling the bacteria or its spores. TB usually affects the lungs but can also affect other organs such as the kidneys, the brain or the spine. *Mycobacterium bovis* can also cause a similar set of symptoms. Eating beef or unpasteurised dairy products is responsible for the spread of this bacterium. We shall focus on *M. tuberculosis* in this brief account of the disease.

What are the symptoms of TB?

The signs and symptoms of the disease include weight loss, coughing and chest pain, blood in sputum, loss of appetite, nausea, fever, chills, night sweats and a pale drawn appearance. Symptoms of TB when it infects organs other than the lungs depend on the organ infected.

The study of tuberculosis illustrates vividly the influence of the environment on the incidence of the disease. Of course you need to come into contact with the bacterium to develop the disease but not everyone who comes into contact with the bacterium does so. In fact you can have a latent infection without developing the disease at all.

Latent TB Infection

People with latent TB infection have *M. tuberculosis* in their bodies but the bacteria are not active. These people do not have any symptoms and cannot transmit the disease to others. They may develop the disease in the future and may be prescribed treatment to prevent this.

TB disease

People who are infected and develop the disease of TB have active bacteria in their bodies that are multiplying and destroying (lung) tissue. They are capable of spreading the disease. The coughing caused by being infected with active bacteria facilitates the spread of the disease by launching bacteria into the environment where another person can inhale them. These bacteria can also be rendered airborne by sneezing, singing or just speaking.

Not only are live bacteria rendered airborne but also spores of the bacteria – these are resistant to the drying effects of the environment and can survive for extended periods of time in bedding, soft furnishings, clothing, etc. Left untreated a person with TB disease of the lungs infects, on average, 10–15 people every year. The risk of someone acquiring the infection depends on the nature and duration of their exposure (see Table 1).

Table 1 TB risk from contact with an infected person

Nature of contact	Risk of infection
None known	1 in 100 000
Casual social contact	1 in 100 000
School or workplace	1 in 50 to 1 in 3
Bar, social club	Up to 1 in 10
Dormitory	1 in 5
Home	1 in 3
Nursing home	1 in 20
Source: *New England Journal of Medicine* (2003); 348: 1256–66 cited in Department of Health (2004b).	

Activity 4

Using Table 1 suggest what other factors may contribute to the incidence of TB.

Aetiology

Aetiology means the study of the causes of disease. The cause of TB is of course *M. tuberculosis* – but is it that simple? Latent TB infection illustrates that you can have *M. tuberculosis* and not suffer from the disease. What else therefore influences the incidence of TB?

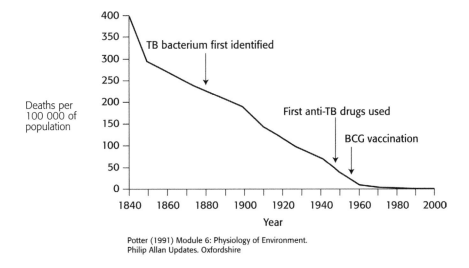

Potter (1991) Module 6: Physiology of Environment.
Philip Allan Updates. Oxfordshire

Figure 8 The death rate from tuberculosis in England and Wales (Potter, 1991)

Activity 5

The antibiotic streptomycin was first introduced in 1944 and the BCG vaccination in 1950.

Using a pencil, draw a vertical line up from both of these dates in Figure 8. Where each line meets the curve draw a horizontal line to the y-axis. What conclusions can you draw?

There are many other factors that contribute to the incidence of TB:

- overcrowding;
- damp, poorly ventilated housing;
- malnutrition;
- drug use;
- HIV/AIDS – in England at least three per cent of people with TB are estimated to be HIV positive and the percentage is higher in London.
  (DoH, 2004d)

Activity 6

Can you give one reason why each of these factors could influence the incidence of TB?

Treatment and prevention

Treatment of TB requires a six-month course of a combination of three or four drugs. These include:

- isoniazid;
- rifampicin;
- pyrazinamide;
- ethambutol.

Failure to complete the prescribed course of drugs as directed can lead to the development of the disease again and/or the evolution of drug-resistant strains of the bacterium.

> Care of people with TB needs to be orientated around helping them take their treatment consistently over the long period of time it takes to achieve a cure.
>
> (DoH, 2004d)

Prevention

Vaccination (BCG vaccine) is with a weakened strain of *M. bovis*. It was developed in France and introduced into the UK in the 1950s. The bacteria are alive but weakened so that they do not cause the disease. The surface antigens are intact and stimulate an immune response and the subsequent production of memory cells, and therefore immunity.

MDR-TB and XDR-TB

Multidrug-resistant TB (MDR-TB) is defined as a strain of TB that is resistant to both rifampicin and isoniazid. Treatment involves a five-drug regimen for an extended period of time. XDR-TB or extensive drug-resistant TB is also resistant to three or more of the six classes of second-line drugs. The first case of XDR-TB reported in the UK was in March 2008. A Somalian man in his 30s was in isolation in a Glasgow hospital. Treatment takes 12–18 months and costs more than £100 000 per patient. XDR-TB first came to public attention in 2006, when a cluster of cases was reported in South Africa. All 53 patients were HIV positive and 52 of them died within 25 days (**www.guardian. co.uk/society/2008/mar/21/health/print**).

ANTIBIOTICS

The development of resistance to antibiotics is one of the main challenges facing the health care professions today. It therefore requires us to consider what antibiotics are, what they are used for and how they work. The word antibiotic literally means 'against life' and, in particular, against prokaryotic or bacterial life. The term originally referred to substances produced by fungi or bacteria that killed other species of bacteria. Today the term antibiotic is used to refer to anything that kills microbes.

It is important to note that antibiotics do not kill viruses. Antibiotics work by disrupting the physiology or ultrastructure of the prokaryote. As discussed above, viruses do not have their own physiology and share very few similarities with the ultrastructure of a prokaryote. However, there are antiviral agents that target specific viral enzymes and work by slowing the normal viral reproduction cycle. For example, azidothymidine (AZT) works by inhibiting some of the enzymes needed to replicate the HIV virus but, unfortunately, side effects limit the size of the dose that can be administered.

Alexander Fleming famously discovered penicillin in 1928 when he noticed that a mould was producing a substance that was killing the bacteria he was trying to culture. Many more antibiotics have been discovered from soil microbes and many more have been synthesised by scientists. Antibiotics can either kill bacteria and are termed **bacteriocidal** or they can inhibit the growth of bacteria and are termed **bacteriostatic**. Some antibiotics will affect a wide range of different bacterial species and are termed **broad spectrum** while others affect a much narrower range of bacteria and are termed **narrow spectrum** antibiotics.

How do antibiotics work?

Different antibiotics work in different ways – the following are some examples.

Inhibiting cell wall synthesis

Bacteria cells, unlike human cells, have a cell wall. This prevents the cell from bursting when water enters the bacterium. If this cell wall is weakened by the action of an antibiotic then the cell will burst and die. Penicillin works in this way.

Disrupting the cell membrane

Bacterial and fungal cell membranes differ in composition from human cell membranes. Some antibiotics target this difference and destroy or damage the membrane, which allows the cell contents to leak out and the bacteria or fungal cell then dies. Polymyxins and nystatin work this way on bacteria and fungal cells respectively.

Inhibition of cellular biochemistry

The chemical reactions required for bacterial multiplication and for the production of vital proteins are inhibited by a range of antibiotics. For example, rifampicin and the tetracyclines work in this way.

What is antibiotic resistance and how does it evolve?

If an antibiotic no longer works against a species or strain of bacteria then that species or strain is said to be resistant. How does this evolve? Within a population of bacteria there will be genetic variation in the same way that within a group of humans there is variation in height, hair colour, eye colour, skin colour, etc. In bacteria these variable characteristics may include the ability to resist the effects of a particular antibiotic because the bacteria have evolved and have developed the ability to produce a particular **enzyme** that breaks down the antibiotic (see ESBLs on page 27). When that antibiotic is applied only those bacteria that produce this enzyme will survive and will therefore have less competition for nutrients and, as a result, will reproduce and thrive. When they reproduce the genes that control the production of the particular enzyme are duplicated and the resulting population is resistant.

However, there is another way in which a population of bacteria can become resistant. At the beginning of this chapter we mentioned that bacteria could pass their genes horizontally as well as vertically, that is they can transfer genes from individual to individual. Therefore a resistant bacterium with the gene that controls the production of the enzyme is able to pass a copy of this gene to another bacterium. This bacterium can then pass a copy to another as can the original one, and so on. So a population of bacteria with only one or two resistant individuals to start with can very rapidly become totally resistant.

Why do resistant strains evolve in health care settings?

Antibiotics are being used all of the time in health care settings so to be resistant to the antibiotic is a real advantage for bacteria and therefore only resistant bacteria will survive.

Extended-spectrum β lactamases (ESBLs)

Extended-spectrum β lactamases are enzymes produced by several species of bacteria that break down antibiotics such as the cephalosporins and penicillin. Therefore any bacteria that can produce these enzymes are resistant to a range of antibiotics. So ESBLs are not the bacteria but are enzymes produced by a range of bacterial species that prevent antibiotics killing that bacterium. The gene for ESBL can be passed from bacterium to bacterium via horizontal transfer, thereby spreading resistance.

E. coli and *Klebsiella* species have been identified as producing ESBLs. Since 2003 there has been a marked increase in the incidence of ESBLs mainly due to new strains of bacteria that produce a particular type of ESBL, the CTX-M type, which is able to break down a wider range of antibiotics (**www.hpa.org.uk/infections/topics_az/esbl/default.htm**).

PARASITES

How does a parasite differ from a pathogen? Many would argue that a pathogen is indeed a parasite; however, we are going to make a distinction. A parasite can be considered as an organism that lives on or in a host and gains a nutritional advantage from this relationship, while the host suffers a disadvantage (Indge, 2003).

Parasites include organisms such as round worms, tape worms, ticks, fleas, etc. Many of us have experienced nits or head lice, either suffering infestation ourselves as children or combing them out of our own children's hair. Head lice are parasites – they live on us and feed on our blood. They gain a nutritional advantage (our blood) and we suffer a disadvantage (loss of blood, itching). Head lice are small insects – **Pediculus capitis.** They are found in the hair of children and their families. Children of the ages 3–11 and their families are infected most often (**www.cdc.gov/licehead/fact-sheet.htm**). Personal hygiene at school or at home has no influence on the incidence of head lice infestation. Nits are transmitted by direct contact with someone else who is infested and occasionally by contact with the combs, brushes or bedding of someone who is infested. Adults lay their eggs (the nits) at the base of hairs near the scalp. These hatch into nymphs after 8–9 days, which then mature into adult lice after another 9–12 days. Both nymphs and adults feed on blood from the scalp. The adults can live for up to 30 days on a person's head but will die within one or two days of falling off.

Activity 7

The chain of infection

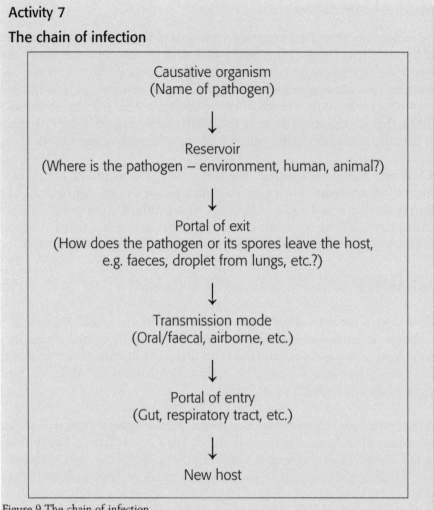

Figure 9 The chain of infection

Construct a chain of infection for TB using the information given in Figure 9. Then research a chain of infection for MRSA.

SUMMARY

The aim of this chapter has been to give you an introduction to some aspects of basic microbiology, cytology and immunology. Particular examples have been used to illustrate aspects of disease and its transmission, as well as some of the other factors that may influence the incidence of disease apart from the presence of the relevant bacterium. The evolution of resistant strains of pathogens is a major challenge to the National Health Service.

Answers to the activities

Activity 1

The answer is 16 777 216. Each bacteria replicates every 20 minutes. So starting with one, after 20 minutes you have 2, both of these replicate to give 4, all 4 replicate to give 8. After 24 replications you have 16 777 216.

Activity 2

Your answer is correct if you can use it to remember survive, penetrate, reproduce, resist and damage in that order.

Activity 3

Vaccines that infer active immunity contain either:

• pure antigen derived from the relevant pathogen;
• dead pathogen with intact antigen;
• attenuated or weakened pathogen.

All of these will stimulate a specific immune response and the production of memory cells. Some vaccines contain antibodies only and will only give immunity until those antibodies break down. This is called passive immunity.

Activity 4

Duration of exposure and the level of intimacy. The size of the room or space in which time is spent with someone who is contagious would also appear to influence the incidence.

Activity 5

1944 – death rate of 50 per 100 000

1950 – death rate of 40 per 100 000

Conclusion – while the introduction of antibiotics reduced the death rate due to TB it was already falling rapidly before this.

Activity 6

- Overcrowding – increased chance of transmission due to close proximity.
- Damp, poorly ventilated housing – increased chance of chest infections due to damp therefore people more susceptible. Same for poor ventilation.
- Malnutrition – compromised immune system.
- Drug use – compromised immune system.
- HIV/AIDS – in England at least 3 per cent of people with TB are estimated to be HIV positive and the percentage is higher in London (DoH, 2004d) – due to a compromised immune system.

Activity 7

TB chain of infection

- *M. tuberculosis*
- Spores in environment/person with TB disease
- Droplets from lungs
- Airborne transmission
- Respiratory tract

MRSA chain of infection

- Methicillin-resistant *Staphylococcus aureus*
- Infected people; infected equipment, e.g. catheters; hands of health care workers
- Faeces/mucous/skin
- Oral/faecal/direct contact
- Wounds/mucous membranes/post-operative

Chapter 2

Infections in the Workplace

In this chapter you will learn about the following:

- HCAIs and 'superbugs' – why are they such a problem?
- Who is at risk and why?
- Hospital-acquired infections prevalent today: a statistical overview, rates of infections in hospitals, care homes and in the community – facts and figures.
- Communicable diseases and public health – TB, flu, legionnaires' disease, etc.
- Effects on patients, care workers and the economy – why does infection prevention and control matter?

HCAI AND SUPERBUGS – WHY ARE THEY SUCH A PROBLEM?

Any infection which has been acquired as a result of a health care procedure or intervention is defined as a health-care associated infection (HCAI or HAI). These infections may be found in hospitals, primary care or community settings such as a client's own home or in residential care.

Confusingly, the press often use the terms HCAIs and 'superbugs' synonymously yet they are not the same thing. HCAIs are any infection acquired in the health care environment but they are not necessarily 'superbugs'. Superbugs are pathogens that have become resistant to treatment and they are present both in the health care environment and in the wider community. So HCAIs can become superbugs given the right conditions (see antibiotic resistance on page 26).

Despite the advances in modern care and medical technology the simple fact remains: people still die from infective disorders that can be prevented by standard measures. In fact, the Chief Medical Officer's report *Winning Ways: Working Together to Reduce Healthcare Associated Infection in England* (DoH, 2003c) estimates that 15 to 20 per cent of HCAI is preventable. (The report may be found at **www.dh.gov.uk/en/**

Publicationsandstatistics/Publications/PublicationsPolicyAndGuidance
/Browsable/DH_4095070 (accessed 6 August 2008).)

Activity 1

Download this report from the Department of Health website and read 'The Present Position'. Write a summary of the piece identifying the following:

- the six points as outlined in the paper;
- the assumptions about infection control and the evidence;
- the suggested approaches.

(Answers to all relevant activities are given at the end of the chapter.)

The rise of HCAIs as a cause of preventable illness and death has provoked much consternation among care workers and the prevention and control of these infections has become something of a priority today. Historically, we have travelled a long path in terms of understanding the causes of infection but new challenges are present today with the advent of infections that threaten to become largely untreatable, at least with current antibiotics and drugs at our disposal.

Cleanliness certainly has a part to play in the reduction of infection but it is not the only factor. Other factors include the general health and age of the person, the presence of underlying disease and nutritional status. The influence of Florence Nightingale and her reform of the hospitals has been far-reaching and continued to constitute much of the training of nurses even into the 1970s. Damp dusting, asepsis and cleaning of beds and furniture formed a large part of the nurse's daily routine and contributed much to the reduction and even the prevention of infection.

The discovery of pathogens, which we can attribute to people such as Pasteur and Koch, demonstrated that the cause of disease was a more complex issue than was originally thought. Their discoveries put the miasma theory, so prevalent in the late 1800s, to rest after hundreds of years and in its place came the concept that the causes of disease were a far more complex set of circumstances.

At this point it is useful to revisit the chain of infection as discussed in Chapter 1 and revised in Figure 1 below. The host is the person who can be affected by the disease. In particular, some people are more susceptible than others to disease due to the environment in which they live and we will discuss this later. When subjected to the organism these individuals may be more at risk of the disease. It is the breaking of this cycle of infection that is important in the control of disease and infection.

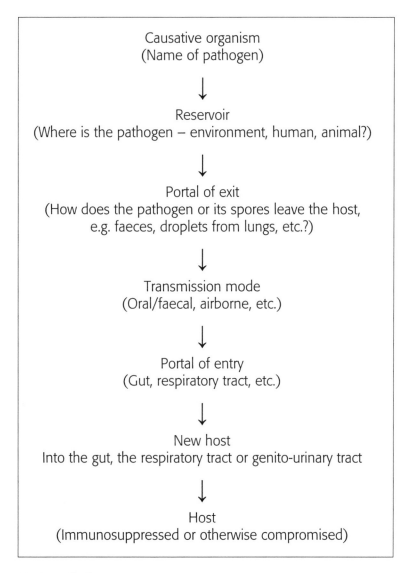

Figure 1 Chain of infection

HCAIs IN TODAY'S HEALTH AND SOCIAL CARE ENVIRONMENTS

Let's now look in more detail at some of the infections we are facing in health care today.

It is possible that the first HCAI on your list will be MRSA or methicillin-resistant *Staphyloccus aureus* but have you also highlighted vancomycin-resistant *enterococci* (**VRE**), *Escherichia coli* or the ESBL or extended-spectrum β lactamases, and the *Clostridium difficile* (C. *diff*) infections? Perhaps you also mentioned TB as well as influenza? Although, in fact, these are not necessarily HCAIs, we will look further at TB and influenza later on in the book as both have become or have the potential to become superbugs.

While we have known about these bacteria for years it is only recently that they have acquired 'superbug' status and the subsequent media reporting has caused alarm for the public and professionals alike. It has encouraged the government to take a more proactive approach to the control of these infections and the Chief Medical Officer has proposed a strategy for combating infectious diseases highlighting the HCAIs and antimicrobial resistance.

It is interesting to note that these types of infections are not new. The concern has been that, although we have always had infections that have been acquired in care settings, they are now on the increase and they are of a nature that is far more difficult to eradicate due to the resistance of the organisms to treatment. Having said that, HCAIs and superbugs are not the same thing, nor are they mutually exclusive as you can acquire a 'superbug' while in a health care setting and in the community.

In the 1940s control of hospital infection was high on the agenda to ensure that susceptible patients in the hospitals were protected in some way. The organisation of control of infection officers and the newly-formed infection control committees addressed the problems occurring back then and, in 1959, the first infection control nurse was appointed. As we noted in our first activity, infection control has now been placed as an essential hospital service because of the increasing problems with highly susceptible patients who, because of multiple factors, have an increased risk of infection.

WHO IS AT RISK AND WHY?

In identifying the 'at risk' patients we can highlight certain general factors and others which may be invoked due to the types of treatment they may be having. These are shown in Table 1.

General factors	Reason
Age	The very young or the very old
Unable to perform personal hygiene tasks	Being dependent upon a carer to provide for hygiene needs
Malnourished	Over or underweight
Disease already present	Underlying conditions such as cancer or diabetes
Loss of mobility	Poor circulation and more prone to pressure sores
Mental state	Confused
Incontinence	Problems with hygiene
Other factors	
Trauma caused by foreign bodies and the effect of treatment	Catheterisation or cannulation as well as traumatic entry into the body of an object
Drugs	Immunosuppressant or cytotoxic drugs reduce immune response
Health conditions	Skin lesions or swelling of limbs as in oedema

Table 1 Factors that influence the acquisition of HCAIs

As Table 1 reveals, some patients are more at risk of acquiring infection and the risk is particularly high when the patient is in hospital or a care setting. This is because they are more likely to be dealt with by a number of staff, treated using equipment and they are exposed to other patients and their visitors, which can all act as a source of infection.

However, as the boundary between in-patient and out-patient care becomes more blurred, with patients being sent home following day-case procedures, the distinction is not as clear. There is now evidence that infections in the community are on the increase because many patients who would originally have had a longer hospital stay are being nursed at home. There is therefore a need to be as vigilant in the community about how we view infection control as there is in the care setting. Consider the following case study which has been adapted from a real case.

Case study 1

Jane Sycamore, a 70-year-old woman, went into her local hospital for an operation to remove a benign tumour from her colon.

The ten-minute procedure went very well and she was returned to the ward and then was discharged home. Her daughter reported that, following her return home, her mother started to feel unwell.

The family tried to have her re-admitted but the bed had been taken, so Mrs Sycamore was removed to a neighbouring hospital. Blood tests confirmed that Mrs Sycamore had MRSA. She later died from septi-caemia.

From your knowledge reflect on the ways in which this patient could have contracted MRSA.

Mrs Sycamore is more than likely to have contracted the condition in the first hospital and special precautions may not have been in place to prevent this happening. We will look at these precautions in more detail later but it is sufficient to say that this early case (2002), high-lighting the MRSA infection, has moved the infection control agenda along a great deal.

Activity 4

What special precautions might you have put into place to prevent Mrs Sycamore's infection?

We will look in depth at the answer to this Activity in Chapter 3 so, in the meantime, save your work and look closely at the figures given below.

It is clear that some people will be more susceptible to infections than others but, with the impact of excellent treatments and care, many people now live much longer. This has affected the national demographic figures and we now see far greater numbers of elderly people in our population, many of whom require additional care in order to keep them healthy and living fulfilled lives. This will, of course, have an effect on the prevalence of HCAIs.

RATES OF INFECTION IN HOSPITALS, CARE HOMES AND THE COMMUNITY – FACTS AND FIGURES

So what are the latest figures and the statistics to demonstrate the prevalence of these infections? Let's look at the three most common infections.

MRSA

The Department of Health published the following figures in 2005 to show the prevalence of MRSA:

- The total number of methicillin-resistant *Staphylococcus aureus* bacteraemias in England in April to September 2005 was 3580. The corresponding figure for the same time period in the previous four years was 3616 (2001), 3584 (2002), 3749 (2003) and 3525 (2004).
- The number of MRSA bacteraemias in the first four complete years of the mandatory recording system were 7247 in 2001/2, 7372 in 2002/3, 7684 in 2003/4 and 7212 in 2004/5.

(Health Protection Agency, 2005a)

This would seem to indicate a stabilisation in the incidence of this particular infection. Government initiatives such as *Essential Steps* (DoH, 2007b) and *Towards Cleaner Hospitals and Lower Rates of Infection* (DoH, 2004e) will be discussed later in the book. National Surveillance Surveys are now carried out every six months and they have confirmed that 9 per cent of patients had an HCAI at the time of the latest survey in 2007.

It is certainly true that the rates of infection vary in hospitals throughout the country and those with more vulnerable patients report higher levels of infection, which is to be expected and in no way reflects their performance. In February of 2008 the National Statistics Office (NSO) published the following figures and graph to show that the deaths from MRSA seemed to have stabilised (see Figure 2).

Number of deaths

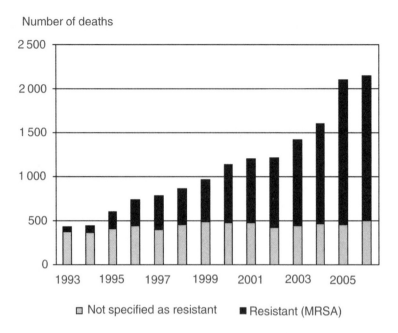

☐ Not specified as resistant   ■ Resistant (MRSA)

Figure 2 Deaths from MRSA 1993–2006 (National Statistics Office, February 2008)

The figure of 1652 deaths from resistant MRSA in 2006 follows the year-on-year increases since 1993 as we can see from the graph in Figure 2. In fact, the report shows that deaths where MRSA was the underlying cause have stabilised and now account for one in three (**www.statistics.gov.uk/ CCI/nugget.asp?ID=1067**). It is apparent that in the older population MRSA is a more prevalent cause of death than in younger age groups with 916 and 417 deaths per million population for males and females respectively in 2006 in the 85 and over age group. So MRSA remains an issue but is seemingly becoming less prevalent.

Furthermore, the NSO has stated that the number of death certificates mentioning *Staphylococcus aureus* has been relatively constant over the period 1993–2006 and deaths from this cause have been highest in the male population with an increase noted between 2005 and 2006. In females the rate went down from 14 to 13 per million population over the same period.

Staphylococcus aureus is carried harmlessly on the skin or in the nose by about 30 per cent of the population and a letter from the Chief Medical Officer in 1996 brought this to the attention of care home owners. The letter stated that while 80 per cent of people acquiring MRSA carry the bacteria harmlessly it is only those patients whose resistance is impaired who may go on to get an infection. Care home owners were urged not to be alarmed by the figures from hospitals and the letter went on to say that MRSA only poses a minor threat to those people in care establishments.

The Department of Health's view is that the fact that a person has MRSA is not a reason to prevent their admission to a suitable home or to prevent them mixing socially with other residents.

(Department of Health, 1996)

So we seem to be getting control of the MRSA phenomenon and figures from the National Statistics Office show a stabilisation of the threat. However, the emergence of new and different strains of infections has become more worrying.

C. *difficile*

Activity 5

In Chapter 1 you were asked to construct a chain of infection for MRSA. See if you can recall it now. Now produce a chain of infection for *C. difficile*. Use the case study shown on page 19 and the information below to help you.

An emerging problem is the incidence in our hospitals and care homes of the bacteria that, although found in the large bowel of less than 5 per cent of the healthy adult population, is now presenting a threat to the health care community. The *Clostridium difficile* bacterium is a major cause of antibiotic associated diarrhoea and colitis. It is part of the Clostridium family of bacteria and these also cause tetanus, gas gangrene and botulism. Patients treated with broad spectrum antibiotics are at greatest risk of C. *difficile* associated disease. Risks become higher when the patient is elderly or has a serious underlying illness that compromises their immune system, or they have a protracted stay in health care settings. Recent gastrointestinal surgery also increases the risk of infection (**www.statistics.gov.uk/cci/ nugget.asp?ID=1735).**

Identified in the 1930s, this bacterium emerged in the 1970s as the cause of diarrhoea and colitis following antibiotic therapy. An outbreak at Stoke Mandeville Hospital raised concerns due to the propensity of the bacteria to spread between patients quite readily and the severity of the symptoms caused, sometimes leading to fatal consequences from peritonitis and perforated bowel. This led to C. *difficile* becoming part of the mandatory surveillance programme for health-care associated infections in 2004.

Statistics from the C. *diff* support website show that you are 2.3 times more likely to die of C. *difficile* than MRSA in England and Wales and C. *difficile* has been linked to:

1214 deaths in 2001
1428 deaths in 2002
1788 deaths in 2003
2247 deaths in 2004
3807 deaths in 2005

(www.cdiff-support.co.uk)

The data above must be viewed with some caution since it has been made available from a website that has been set up by a support group following the death of a loved one. We therefore turn our attention to the Health Protection Agency (HPA) and their data. Reporting on the number of cases annually, the HPA show an increase in cases due to improved testing and better reporting systems. From less than 1000 cases reported in the1990s the number of cases has increased to 22 000 in 2002, 28 000 in 2003 and 44 488 in 2004. A marked increase is shown which is quite alarming and the NSO has confirmed these figures and published the graph in Figure 3 to show the increase.

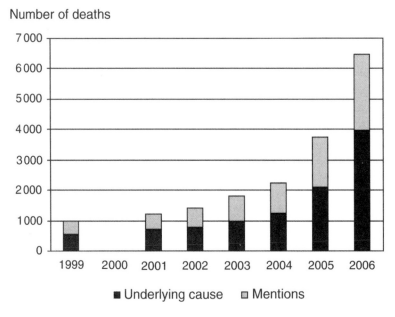

Figure 3 The number of death certificates mentioning C. *difficile* and recording C. *difficile* as the underlying cause of death in England and Wales (NB there is no data available for 2000) (**www.statistics.gov.uk/cci/nugget.asp?ID=1735**, accessed 28 February 2008)

It therefore seems that the number of deaths from this particular infection has increased each year from 1999 resulting in 6480 deaths in 2006, which represents a 72 per cent increase from 2005. Again it is the older age groups who are more at risk with both males and females suffering equally (**www.statistic.gov.uk/cci/nugget.asp?ID=1735**, accessed February 2008).

E. coli and ESBL

With the increases in the number of infections reported from C. *difficile* in 2003 there also emerged a further threat to the population by way of a strain of E. *coli* that produce extended-spectrum ß lactamases or ESBL. Microbiologists from the South East and West Midlands reported the emergence of infections caused by cephalosporin-resistant strains of E. *coli*. These were being seen in high numbers in the local community with patients over the age of 60 contracting urinary infections. Some of these patients had previously been catheterised. These types of bacteria resist the action of antibiotics by producing an enzyme which destroys the antibiotic. Infection usually occurs in the urinary tract but can also infect wounds and may become blood-borne.

GRE

The total number of reports of clinically significant GRE (glycopeptide-resistant enterococci) bacteraemia in England between October 2003 and September 2004 was 620 but there has been a year-on-year increase in the numbers between the years 1994 and 2004, with numbers in this decade more than doubling. There were 8640 cases in 1994 increasing to 17 416 cases in 2004. The alarming feature of this particular bacterium is its ability to evolve into an organism that is resistant to more antibiotics each year.

COMMUNICABLE DISEASES AND PUBLIC HEALTH

The new so-called 'superbugs' continue to pose a threat to our health but what of the older types of infections that we have been able to control to a certain extent? Let's now turn our attention to the pathogens that still pose a considerable threat to our lives despite major advances in technology and medicine.

Tuberculosis

The World Health Organization (WHO) has highlighted that tuberculosis remains a major cause of death worldwide. This may surprise us since in this country it has largely been eradicated. However, in 2005, 8.8 million new cases worldwide were reported resulting in 1.6 million deaths. In fact, in March 2008 a confirmed case of the most resistant strain XDR-TB was reported in Birmingham.

Tuberculosis is a preventable and curable airborne infectious disease and individuals ill with TB bacteria in their lungs can infect others through coughing. If detected early and treated, individuals can expect to become non-infectious and will eventually be cured. It is, however, the multi drug-resistant TB (MDR-TB), extensive drug-resistant TB (XDR-TB) and HIV-associated TB strains that cause issues within the health care system (see Chapter 1 for more information on TB).

WHO is working to reduce the burden of TB and aims to halve TB deaths and prevalence by 2015, through its *Stop TB Strategy* and by supporting the *Global Plan to Stop TB* (WHO, 2006a and b).

In England, Wales and Northern Ireland cases of tuberculosis have increased by 10.8 per cent from 7321 cases reported in 2004 to 8113 in 2005. These figures were released by the Health Protection Agency and were the largest increase since 1999. The age profile of those prone to suffer from TB is shown in Figure 4.

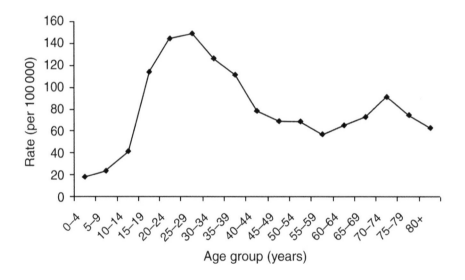

Figure 4 Tuberculosis rates in non-UK born persons by age group, England, Wales and Northern Ireland, 2006 *Source*: Enhanced Tuberculosis Surveillance, Labour Force Survey population estimates, as at 20/07/2007. *Prepared by*: Health Protection Agency Centre for Infections.

London reported the highest notification rate of tuberculosis in 2004 with 34.8 notifications per 100 000 people living in the region. This is more than twice the second highest rate of 16.4 in the West Midlands. Northern Ireland had the lowest notification rate of 4.3 per 100 000 of the population. The introduction of the WHO surveillance system, which provides more detailed information about the patterns of TB, revealed that London also had the highest number of cases in 2005 (43 per cent), increasing from 3129 in 2004 to 3479 in 2005.

It appears that in many areas there has been a growth in the incidence of TB in the ten years prior to 2004. According to NSO figures the rate in the East of England has increased by over 60 per cent although, at 7.6 per 100 000 population in 2004, the rate remained below that of 12.1 for the UK as a whole. In the North West the 588 cases in 2004 rose to 757 cases in 2005. The East Midlands had 443 cases in 2004 and this increased to 556 in 2005. The East of England fared marginally better with the lowest number of cases being shown as 395 in 2004 increasing to 483 in 2005. The North East and Northern Ireland saw a decrease in cases with 149 in 2004 compared with 134 in 2005 and 81 cases in 2004 compared with 76 in 2005 respectively. In Wales the number of cases remained the same at 191.

The Indian, Pakistani and Bangladeshi ethnic group made up the highest proportion of cases reported in 2005 (3075 cases compared to 2574 in 2004) followed by the Black African group (1932 cases compared to 1766 to 2004) and the White group (1721 in 2005 compared to 1729 in 2004).

This last point might suggest that people from other countries have brought the disease into the UK. However, as only 22 per cent of these groups arrived within the last two years the suggestion is that a combination of the disease developing in individuals who may already have been infected and new infections acquired in the UK is the more likely reason for the increase. Travel to other countries where TB is common may also be a factor (**www.hpa.org.uk/infections/topics_az/tb/data_menu.htm**).

Of course, any increase in a disease that is likely to develop into a multi-resistant strain and that could cause the deaths of thousands of patients in our health care system is of concern to all health professionals. The government and the Department of Health are therefore rightly concerned and are putting into place systems to monitor the situation. The Health Protection Agency works with health professionals to improve the prevention and control of TB. Their activities include the surveillance and diagnosis of TB, advice on how to manage outbreaks and investigation into the clinical, social and environmental factors that are associated with such an infection.

Activity 6

Visit the HPA website at: **www.hpa.org.uk/infections/**

This website will give you a valuable insight into the data available on all major concerns in health care. Familiarise yourself with the website and read about the major diseases. Look at the information on influenza and then read the next section.

Influenza – the ever present pandemic threat

In the winter months we usually see reports of an increase in many respiratory and circulatory deaths and influenza is often thought to be implicated. In 2006–7 influenza was below baseline levels and not as high as the epidemic activity reported in 1999–2000 according to HPA figures.

Infection is caused by one of a group of viruses called the orthomyxo-viruses. The influenza virus was first identified in 1933. There are three types of virus, A, B and C, with type A causing most epidemics and infecting birds and animals. The subsequent respiratory illness is characterised by headaches, fever and sore throat together with aching muscles and joints. Bronchitis and secondary bacterial pneumonia are the most common complications of influenza and hospitalisation may be required, particularly for the elderly, asthmatics and those in poor health, where the disease is life-threatening.

History books cite the 'Spanish flu' epidemic of 1918 as causing the deaths of more people than the First World War. Since that time there have been further epidemics and the emergence of variant strains of the disease is threatening to produce pandemic activity. A pandemic is a global epidemic and occurs when a new virus appears against which we have no immunity. This can lead to enormous numbers of deaths. Our international transport system around the globe as well as the rise in population in urban areas leading to overcrowded conditions means that influenza outbreaks can quickly spread across the globe.

The history of influenza

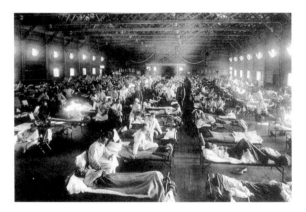

Figure 5 Emergency military hospital during the influenza epidemic in 1918, Camp Funston, Kansas, United States Image courtesy of the National Museum of Health and Medicine, Armed Forces Institute of Pathology, Washington, DC, United States. Reproduced under the Creative Commons Attribution 2.5 License. *Source*: **http://dx.doi.org/10.1371/journal.-pbio.0040050**.

Spanish flu 1918–19

The 'Spanish flu' (1918–19) (so called because the pandemic received greater attention in Spain than in the rest of Europe) was caused by a severe and deadly strain of the H1N1 subtype of influenza A. While the origin of the pandemic is unknown it was thought to have started with the deployment of soldiers throughout Europe. Travelling from North America through Europe and into North Africa the illness then reached India, China and New Zealand.

Although efforts were made to contain the disease the fatalities were enormous and many institutions were closed to try to prevent further transmission. Isolation, disinfection and the prevention of public meetings was called for to try to stop the spread.

Asian flu 1957–58

The 'Asian flu' of 1957–58 was an outbreak of avian flu that started in China and spread worldwide that same year. Within six months, the pandemic spread throughout the world. In Europe the epidemic, which coincided with the September return to school, was concentrated in school children, but in the UK it was the elderly who suffered the most mortalities.

A second wave of infection was observed early in 1958, and caused high rates of illness and increased fatalities. Forty to fifty per cent of people were affected by the two waves of the disease, of which 25–30 per cent experienced disease. An estimate of the mortality rate was over one million people.

Hong Kong flu (1968)

In 1968 an outbreak of flu began in China, spreading to Hong Kong that same month and from there it spread rapidly across the world. In just two weeks 500 000 cases were reported in Hong Kong alone. In 1968 the WHO warned about the emergence of a possible pandemic and South East Asia reported a rapid spread over the next six months. The US marines returning from the Vietnam War took the virus to the USA in September 1968 and by December the illness was widespread. Morbidity and mortality were as high as in the 1957–58 pandemic. In the UK the epidemic began in December. Estimates of the number of victims of the 1968 pandemic show a range of between 1 and 3 million fatalities, of which over 30 000 were from the UK.

TOWER HAMLETS COLLEGE
POPLAR HIGH STREET
LONDON
E14 0AF

So with three major pandemics to learn from what do we do in this country to prevent such a disease from happening again?

The prevention and control of influenza

The monitoring and recording of the incidence of seasonal flu in the UK is the responsibility of the Health Protection Agency and the information gathered is used to guide the development of policies for protecting the UK population from influenza. Working in tandem with Health Protection Scotland, the CDSC Northern Ireland, the National Public Health Service for Wales, the Royal College of General Practitioners, NHS Direct and the Department of Primary Care at Nottingham University the data is collected and distributed nationwide.

A seasonal summary is produced tabling the respiratory and viral activity for given periods. In 2006–7 the summary reported 38 outbreak reports of influenza-like illness across England and Wales with the majority (53 per cent) arising in schools and, of the 13 outbreaks confirmed as influenza, 12 were typed as influenza A.

Despite the seemingly low levels of influenza-type activity you are no doubt aware of the threat of so-called 'bird flu' which has cropped up in various countries around the globe. Avian flu, a highly contagious disease found in many bird species, is caused by the type A influenza virus and is a notifiable disease. A serious outbreak occurred in the Netherlands in 2003 and spread to Belgium and Germany resulting in the slaughter of more than 28 million poultry. Since that time there have been a number of reported cases throughout the world leading to a frenzy of media reporting about this relatively new strain of the influenza virus.

The HPA and the WHO are aware of the need to prepare for a further pandemic. With outbreaks of influenza in animals and birds, together with annual outbreaks in humans, the chances of a pandemic multiply due to the merging of animal and human influenza viruses. It is felt that the occurrence of the next pandemic is just a matter of time (HPA, 2005b). This has led to the HPA taking steps to improve the UK's preparedness for a future influenza pandemic. To this end there has been the development of information and guidance, emergency planning, exercises, training, laboratory work and regional, national and international liaison.

Global surveillance of influenza via a network of 112 National Influenza Centres monitoring influenza activity reports the emergence of 'unusual' influenza viruses. This rapid detection of influenza outbreaks and the subsequent isolation of possible pandemic viruses is the key to preventing the occurrence of a future pandemic which could kill millions of people worldwide.

The Centers for Disease Control and Prevention in Atlanta USA predict that if a pandemic happened today it is likely to result in 2 to 7.4 million deaths globally, with a demand for 134–233 million out-patient visits and 1.5–5.2 million hospital admissions.

Activity 7

Construct a chain of infection to show how an outbreak of influenza might start in a residential care home.

It is of concern that the outbreak of a pandemic is thought by some health care professionals to be inevitable and to that end we need to be vigilant in preparing for such an occurrence. The *Infection Control in Community Settings* document, which has been prepared by the National Public Health Service for Wales (see Activity 8), is a useful text to become acquainted with. It identifies what to do if flu is suspected in your clients in the care setting and details how we might all deal with an outbreak of flu in the community. Using cards, which can be displayed easily in the health care setting, it outlines procedures for preventing the spread of infection.

Activity 8

You are advised to look at the document *Infection Control in Community Settings* now by accessing the website **www2.nphs. wales.nhs.uk:8080/FluPandemicDocs.nsf** and clicking on 'Infection control in the community practice'.

Legionnaires' disease

The *Guardian* newspaper in 2007 published the following reports of the outbreaks of legionnaires' disease.

'Pirbright worker contracts legionnaires' disease'
'Cruise passengers test positive for legionnaires' disease'
'Patient who overcame leukemia killed by a dirty hospital shower'
'Legionnaires' disease deaths blamed on flaws in council policy'

Our final communicable disease, legionnaires' disease, is, again, likely to affect middle-aged or older people, smokers, heavy drinkers, people with respiratory diseases or those with impaired immunity and it produces symptoms similar to those of flu.

The legionella bacterium *L. pneumophila* is found naturally in environmental water sources but, within a building, it can colonise manufactured water systems and rapidly spreads to cooling tower systems, hot and cold water systems, and other plant that use or store water.

Although a fairly uncommon disease, 40 different strains of the legionella bacterium have been discovered and it can cause a potentially fatal form of pneumonia in immuno-compromised patients. Hospitalised patients are therefore vulnerable to such an outbreak. One such case was that of Daryl Eyles, 37, who contracted legionnaires' disease from a dirty shower head while recovering in hospital from cancer.

The *Guardian* in 2007 reported the figures for legionnaires' disease as being around 300 to 350 cases in England and Wales each year with the incidence having risen sharply in recent years. There were 163 cases between January and June in 2007, compared with 120 in the same period in 2006 and 105 in 2005.

As a possible hospital acquired infection we need to be aware of the potential for vulnerable patients to be subject to conditions that could lead to infection. Organisations, including hospitals, that operate man-made water systems must comply with regulations requiring them to maintain and clean them properly. This means that the water must be treated and the system cleaned regularly (Health and Safety Executive, 2003).

THE EFFECTS OF HCAIs ON SERVICE USERS AND THE ECONOMY

The cost to the NHS of treating HCAIs and, indeed, the cost to society as a whole is a complex issue. In terms of the financial burden to the NHS, this can be shown by the monetary expense of treating patients with infections. However, a far more pressing concern has to be the effects on the patients/clients themselves and the effects on the primary care services when patients leave the hospital setting.

A study by Plowman *et al.* in 1999 set out to describe the effects with the specific objectives of determining the costs to the secondary, primary and community health sectors, patients and carers, and the economy as a whole. Four groups of patients were identified:

- those without infections during their hospital stay and afterwards;
- those who had no infection during in-patient stay but reported symptoms following discharge;
- patients with one or more infections noted while in-patients but not reporting symptoms when discharged;
- patients who had one or more HCAIs during the in-patient phase and reported symptoms following discharge.

Patients who had one or more HCAIs during their hospital stay on average incurred costs to the health services of £3145 more than those who had no infection. This was a percentage increase of 2.9 per cent. The graph in Figure 6 shows how these costs are distributed.

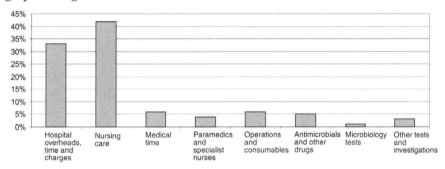

Figure 6 The percentage increase in costs incurred to the health services as a result of patients with one or more HCAIs Data adapted from report by Plowman *et al.*, (1999).

The type of infection the patient had also had an impact on cost. Urinary infections incurred an extra cost of £1327, which represents a 1.8 per cent increase, whereas patients with lower respiratory tract, skin and wound infections were more likely to attract an additional cost of between £1618 and £2398 per patient equivalent to a 2–2.5 per cent increase. In cases where a blood-borne infection such as septicaemia was acquired the cost rocketed to an additional £5397 per patient. On average the length of stay for infected patients amounted to 11 extra days in hospital. This varied with the infection site and type.

Of course the cost implications are not confined to hospital stays. When the patients were discharged to the community an increase in cost to the primary care services was noted in the study. Personal cost to the patient was measured by the impact of the time it took for resumption of normal daily activity and, in some cases, the return to employment, all of which saw a percentage increase in time. Overall the cost to the health system is phenomenal. Plowman *et al.* report that:

HAIs were estimated to cost the NHS in England £986.36 million annually. Of this aggregate cost, £930.62 million was estimated to have been incurred during the patients' hospital stay and £55.74 million post discharge.

(Plowman *et al.*, 1999: 13)

These costs represent 9.1 per cent of the annual NHS budget. Interestingly, infections of the urinary tract, although relatively inexpensive to treat, represented the highest incidence of infection and therefore cost more per annum to treat than other infections. In terms of days lost through infection an additional 8.7 million days were taken to resume normal activity.

The effects on the budget are easy to ascertain. A reduction in the prevalence of the infection rate would pay dividends in terms of money saved to the NHS as well as reducing the impact on patients and the economy as a whole. Money spent on prevention has therefore become a more attractive option to the government and, as such, we have seen further moves to increase the budget for this agenda.

The impact of infection within our hospitals and in the community is an issue for all concerned. It is evidently on the increase and is costing the health care system millions of pounds a year. We now turn our attention in the next chapter to the more pressing issue of the attempt to reduce the impact of infection by the use of standard or universal precautions.

SUMMARY

- The influence of Florence Nightingale's reform of hospitals was far-reaching and contributed much to the reduction and even the prevention of infection. However, although cleanliness has played a part in the reduction of infection, it is not the only factor. Other factors include the general health and age of the person, the presence of underlying disease and nutritional status. The emergence in the twentieth century of HCAIs and 'superbugs' has led to far-reaching plans on the part of health professionals to address the emerging problem.
- HCAIs were estimated to cost the NHS in England £986.36 million annually and also affect quality of life.
- The communicable diseases TB, flu and legionnaires' disease have been a part of our lives for hundreds of years but have proved difficult to control and are likely to affect our lives in future with the emergence of drug-resistant forms and the threat of pandemics emerging at any time.

The control of disease is therefore of timely concern to all health professionals and in the following chapters we shall look at how the government and the World Health Organisation are addressing the problem.

Answers to the activities

Activity 1

The six points as outlined in the paper are:

- Infection of in-patients is common and occasionally life-threatening.
- The UK does not perform well in its infection control procedures and while the problem is worldwide we are performing less well than other European countries.
- There is inconsistency in the use of evidence-based countermeasures of effectiveness being implemented in hospitals.
- Antibiotic resistance is worsening and making infections difficult to treat.
- The emergence of 'superbugs' such as MRSA, vancomycin-resistant enterococci and penicillin-resistant *Streptococcus pneumoniae* are posing very high risks.
- Past emphasis on surveillance has meant that the good information on infection control has bypassed the clinical teams and patients.

The assumptions about infection control and the evidence are:

- Hand washing is vitally important in preventing the spread of infection and the failure of staff to do so between patients is due to laziness and carelessness.
- Punishment when staff fail to carry out the procedures is needed.

The evidence is:

- The barriers to hand washing have been identified as the following:
  - lack of knowledge among care staff of guidelines;
  - inadequate facilities;
  - lack of time;
  - lack of hand-washing agents;
  - the need for good leadership, high-quality information and a change in the culture.

The suggested approaches are:

- Commitment from senior managers to change the culture.
- Make health-care associated infections an indicator of quality and safety.
- Apply measures known to reduce risks.
- Enable the provision of good-quality information for public and patients as well as clinical staff so that risks are transparent.

Activity 5

- *Clostridium difficile*.
- Infected people/infected equipment, e.g. catheters, hands of health care workers, patients or residents may have been in contact with patients or staff in the ward carrying the bacteria.
- Faeces/mucous/skin. Poor hand washing techniques by staff or the use of dirty equipment may carry the bacterium to the patient.
- Oral/faecal/direct contact.
- Wounds/mucous membranes/post-operative.

Activity 7

- Causative organism – orthomyxoviruses.
- Reservoir – environment and bird/animal populations.
- Portal of exit – respiratory droplets from respiratory tract.
- Transmission – airborne.
- Portal of entry – respiratory tract.

Chapter 3

Preventing and Controlling Infection: The Law, Policy and Standards

In this chapter you will learn about some of the legal, political, regulatory and guidance instruments, resources and evidence that have been produced to help to prevent and control infection. The documents, policies, etc. referred to in this chapter will include:

- The advent of clinical governance and its impact on policy
- Health and Safety at Work Act 1974
- Standard Universal Precautions
- Commission for Health Care Audit and Inspection (CHAI)
- Commission for Health Improvement
- The Health Act 2006
- The Public Health (Infectious Diseases) Regulations 1988
- Hazardous Waste Regulations 2005
- Skills for Health and Skills for Care workforce competencies
- Health Care Commission Standards
- EPIC Guidelines: **www.epic.tvu.ac.uk**
- NICE
- Department of Health – *Essential Steps to Safe, Clean Care*
- RCN and NMC – *Essential Skills Clusters, Good Practice in Infection Prevention and Control*

You will also cover the Skills for Care Knowledge Set on Infection Prevention and Control item 3:
3. Legislation relevant to infection prevention and control.
  3.1 Understand the legislation, regulations and guidance that govern infection prevention and control.
  3.2 Understand the organisations, policies and procedures with regard to infection prevention and control.

INTRODUCTION

In Chapter 2 we learned that the cost to the NHS of HCAIs runs into millions of pounds per year. Notwithstanding the cost, there is also the issue of public confidence in a health service that could compromise the health of vulnerable patients and, as such, there have been a number of initiatives put in place to address the issue of HCAIs.

Care establishments must be safe environments and carers are responsible under the laws of this country to safeguard the individuals in their care. The most important right for an individual in a care setting is to have the right to high standards and good-quality care that is safe. With respect to infection prevention there are a number of laws that care workers need to be aware of. Laws are translated into policy statements that your employer is duty bound to produce and make available to staff. They enable the law to be implemented in practice and clearly describe the commitment of the organisation to the promotion of safe practice in all areas of care work.

CLINICAL GOVERNANCE

The government White Paper entitled *A First Class Service: Quality in the New NHS* (DoH, 1998) outlined the principles of clinical governance and the initiative to put clinical quality at the heart of all NHS and community services business. Some of the principles listed below were clearly already in progress in the NHS setting but this initiative was a way of ensuring that all the practices were brought together and the responsibility for clinical governance became part of the Directorate's role with nursing and medical directors working together. The principles outlined:

- quality improvement for clinical services;
- effective risk management practices including health and safety and controls assurance;
- use of evidence-based practice;
- effective complaints management and the management of any subsequent legal activity;
- the development of continuing professional development for clinical staff;
- the placement of systems to monitor performance of clinical staff and to act when professional practice falls below an accepted standard.

The government stated that this quality change in the NHS was part of a ten-year plan but hoped that after two to three years of implementing such principles changes would be evident. Two bodies were set up to set standards to meet these aims and to monitor their effects. These were the National Institute for Health and Clinical Excellence (NICE) and the Commission for Health Improvement (CHI).

NICE and CHI

The National Institute for Health and Clinical Excellence (NICE) was set up in 1999 to offer advice and guidance on issues relating to the use of new medications and technologies that influence cost-effectiveness and efficiency in health provisions. The three main functions of NICE are:

- to appraise existing and new technology used in the NHS;
- to produce clinical guidelines;
- to develop clinical audit and confidential enquiries.

In Scotland the body most closely resembling the work of NICE is the Scottish Health Technology Assessment Centre (SHTAC).

The Commission for Health Improvement was set up as a statutory body by the 1999 Health Act. Its key aim was to standardise clinical quality throughout the NHS and to reduce the levels of malpractice. The principles outlined for the CHI were:

- to lead on the development of Clinical Governance;
- to conduct national and local reviews of the implementation of NICE guidelines;
- to work with the NHS to identify serious problems and to manage major incidents nationwide. The CHI was largely responsible for monitoring the work of NHS Trusts and to carry our spot checks on Trusts where there are perceived deficits in clinical practice. The Clinical Standards Board is the Scottish equivalent of the CHI.

The Health Care Commission

This was all to change, however, and on 31 March 2004 the Commission for Health Improvement ceased operating and the Health Care Commission (HHC) took over its functions. The new commission is an independent body, 'set up to promote and drive improvement in the quality of healthcare and public health'. It has a role in inspection, information giving and improvement of standards, and lists the following aims on its website:

- to assess the management, provision and quality of NHS health care and public health services;
- to review the performance of each NHS Trust and the award of an annual performance rating;
- to regulate the independent health care sector through registration, annual inspection, monitoring of complaints and enforcement;
- to publish information about the state of health care;

- to consider complaints about NHS organisations that the organisations themselves have not resolved;
- to promote the co-ordination of reviews and assessments carried out by ourselves and others;
- to carry out investigations of serious failures in the provision of health care.

(www.healthcarecommission.org.uk)

So, clearly, this Commission has a far-reaching role in the quality of the care we are involved in and, as such, has certain standards we need to follow.

The Health Care Commission's legal name is the Commission for Healthcare Audit and Inspection (CHAI). It was formed by the Health and Social Care (Community Health and Standards) Act 2003 and launched on 1 April 2004.

While NICE and the CHAI are not specifically dealing with just infection control they do, within their quality remit, have a part to play in ensuring that standards and quality are reached.

Activity 1

- When next in your workplace identify the ways in which clinical governance is impacting upon the work of the department. What evidence do you see of clinical governance making a difference to the practice?
- Talk to senior members of staff and ask about their understanding of the principles and work of NICE and the CHAI.

(Answers to all relevant activities are given at the end of the chapter.)

THE LAW RELATING TO INFECTION PREVENTION AND CONTROL

So what are the legal initiatives that are directly involved in infection prevention and control?

The Health and Safety at Work Act 1974

The Health and Safety at Work Act 1974 is an 'umbrella' act covering a range of legislation relating to the work environment. The Act highlights the responsibility of both the employer and employee with respect to safe standards of practice. All employers have a statutory responsibility to create a safe working environment. Employers have to:

- maintain safe conditions of working with safe equipment;
- provide appropriate equipment and clothing for the job;
- ensure that staff are trained in all aspects of their role;
- provide a written policy about health and safety in the workplace.

Employees have the following responsibilities:

- to co-operate with the employer and take responsibility for their own safety and that of others;
- to attend training;
- to keep records and documents with respect to health and safety.

As part of the Act an employer has to have an organised approach to these specific requirements and this requires that a risk assessment of the environment is carried out. All activities within the particular work setting must be scrutinised and potential and actual risks identified and minimised. With respect to infection control this is a vital part of your work and, as such, you are likely to be trained to follow special procedures in order to reduce the risk to individuals in your care. Carry out the following activity now.

Activity 2

Read the health and safety policy for your care setting and think about the following:

- What are your responsibilities with respect to the Health and Safety at Work Act?
- What mention is made of infection control in the policy?
- Carry out a risk assessment to determine the level of risk with respect to infection control in your work setting. You may find the following headings useful:
  - Step One – look for hazards.
  - Step Two – state who might be at risk and why.
  - Step Three – evaluate the risk.
  - Step Four – record your findings.
  - Step Five – assess the effectiveness of precautions.
- What might you change in order to make your work setting safer?

We will return to this activity in Chapter 5 when further details of risk assessing will be covered.

Standard Universal Precautions

It is likely that your infection control policy as part of the health and safety initiatives in your care setting has detailed the **Standard Universal Precautions**, which are a set of principles that all practitioners in care use to minimise the risk of infection transmission between clients and staff.

In the past we used special infection control measures to ensure that clients known to have infections were not at risk of transmitting the infection to others. It was in the 1980s that the concept of Standard Infection Controls, to be used for all clients, was first recommended by the Centres for Disease Control (CDC) in Atlanta, GA in the United States. It is, of course, not possible to know which patients are infected or carrying blood-borne viruses so, with this in mind, the Advisory Committee on Dangerous Pathogens (ACDP) issued guidelines that were to be applied in all nursing and medical procedures.

'Universal Precautions', as defined by the CDC, were a set of precautions or broad principles that were designed to prevent transmission of human immunodeficiency virus (HIV), hepatitis B virus (HBV), and other blood-borne pathogens when providing any form of health or medical care. Under the Standard Universal Precautions, the blood and body fluids of all patients are considered potentially infectious.

While it is an imperative that care workers consider all patients to be a source of infection the Standard Universal Precautions do not negate the need to isolate certain types of infection. Infections such as those transmitted by droplet or airborne means, such as influenza and tuberculosis, still require isolation nursing techniques to be in place and we will come back to this later.

In some institutions, particularly in the USA, a system of Body Substance Isolation (BSI) has been introduced but the Standard Precautions as we know them have largely incorporated these into the general guidelines we are familiar with.

So, what are we talking about when we are dealing with blood-borne infections? What are the things we are most concerned with? In general Standard Universal Precautions apply to blood, any bodily fluid containing visible blood, semen and vaginal secretions. They can also be applied to tissues and cerebrospinal, synovial, pleural, peritoneal, pericardial and amniotic fluids. They are not applied to faeces, nasal secretions, sputum, sweat, tears, urine or vomit unless they contain visible blood. In the dental setting Standard Universal Precautions do not apply to saliva unless visibly contaminated with blood.

Activity 3

Think back to the risk assessment you carried out in Activity 2. What do you think are or should be contained in the list of Standard Universal Precautions? Make a list and compare it with the items given below.

We expect that at the top of your list you identified hand washing and you would be correct. Also included are the following:

- the use of protective barriers such as gloves, gowns, aprons, masks or protective eyewear;
- laundry management;
- waste management;
- clean environment;
- decontamination of equipment;
- management of exposure to body fluids and blood;
- isolation nursing.

We will be considering the ways in which these precautions are being used in the clinical environment in Chapters 4 and 5.

In short, Standard Universal Precautions involve practices that reduce the risk of exposure of the care worker's skin or mucous membranes to infective materials. It is further recommended that all care workers take precautions to prevent injuries caused by needles, scalpels and other sharp instruments or devices.

One point to note here is that there is not an increased risk of pregnant care workers being more susceptible to infections that are blood-borne but if a care worker were to develop HIV infection during pregnancy, the child would also be put at risk. Because of this pregnant health care workers are urged to be especially familiar with, and strictly adhere to, precautions to minimise the risk of HIV transmission.

Other legislation and government initiatives

Despite the guidelines and principles produced we are still battling infections in our hospitals and care settings. In Part Two of the Health Act of 1999 and 2006 reference is made to the Prevention and Control of Health Care Associated Infections. The Secretary of State was charged with issuing a code of practice relating to infection control and called for the Commission for Health Care Audit and Inspections (CHAI) to conduct reviews and investigations of health care settings. In so doing settings found to be failing with respect to the standards and guidelines are to be issued with improvement notices and recommendations for remedying any problems are to be noted.

Other Acts you may need to be aware of are the Public Health (Infectious Diseases) Regulations 1988, which require the notification of infections to a central board and the reporting of incidences with respect to disease, and, more recently, the Hazardous Waste Regulations 2005. New controls on hazardous waste came into force in England, Wales and Northern Ireland on 16 July 2005 replacing the previous 'Special Waste Regime'. Since that date, most producers of hazardous waste, i.e. waste that might be harmful to our health or the environment, in England and Wales have been required to provide information about their premises to the Environment Agency. In your own care setting you need to be aware of how to dispose of such waste and the penalties for not doing so safely will be clearly referred to in a policy.

> **Activity 4**
>
> Think now about the waste disposal arrangements in your own care setting. How have they changed since 2005 and how do they help with infection control in the work place?

The Department of Health report *The Management and Control of Hospital Acquired Infection in NHS Acute Trusts in England* published in 2000 identified the extent of the problem of health-care associated infections (DoH, 2000b). It noted that at any one time there would be 9 per cent of patients in hospital with infections acquired as a result of their stay. The effects of these infections varied and ranged from prolonged stays in hospital to permanent disability and even, for 5000 patients a year, death. They estimated the cost at £1 billion a year and the price of prevention at £150 million, and determined to make the necessary changes to legislation and practice to bring about a cleaner, safer health service. To this end various initiatives were to be put in place. In addition, the emergence of outbreaks of various diseases, notably Severe Acute Respiratory Syndrome (SARS), the fear of new strains of influenza and the threat of bio-terrorist attacks also ensured that the Department of Health set about raising the profile of infection control in the NHS by commissioning various reports to address the problems.

The following text maps the timeline for the various initiatives developed by the Department of Health:

1998   Report of the House of Lords Select Committee on Science and Technology *Resistance to Antibiotics and other Antimicrobial Agents*.

1999   DoH – *Resistance to Antibiotics and other Antimicrobial Agents*: *Action for the NHS following the Government's Response to the House of Lords Science and Technology Committee Report* (see above) (DoH, 1999a).

2000   DoH – *The Management and Control of Hospital Infection: Action for the NHS for the Management and Control of Infection in Hospitals in England* (DoH, 2000b).

2001   The EPIC Project: developing national evidence-based guidelines for preventing health care associated infections. Phase 1: Guidelines for preventing Hospital Acquired Infections (more of this later in this chapter).

2001   The mandatory surveillance system for serious infections caused by *Staphylococcus aureus* (MRSA) was started.

2002   DoH – *Getting Ahead of the Curve: A Strategy for Combating Infectious Diseases (Including Other Aspects of Health Protections)*.

2003   NICE produced guidelines on the prevention of health care associated infection in primary and community care settings.

2003   DoH – *Winning Ways: Working Together to Reduce Health Care Associated Infection in England* (DoH, 2003c).

So what has been the outcome for the control of infection as a result of these initiatives? Let's look in more detail at each one.

In 2002 the Department of Health published *Getting Ahead of the Curve: A Strategy for Combating Infectious Diseases (Including Other Aspects of Health Protections)*. This paper was followed by the government's White Paper *Saving Lives: A Delivery Programme to Reduce Healthcare-Associated Infection Including MRSA* (DoH, 2005) in which a pledge had been made to address the infectious disease issues by producing strategies which:

- described the nature and scope of the threats posed by infectious disease;
- established priorities for action to combat the present and future threats posed.

It was felt that a broad-based approach to health protection was now needed due to the changing climate posed, not only by emerging infections which had previously been relatively small, but also by the changing climate in the world and the threat of chemical and radiation hazards.

Infectious disease, at the beginning of the twenty-first century, accounted for 41 per cent of the global disease burden and millions of deaths from AIDS/HIV, tuberculosis and malaria were reported each year. While infections as major as these kill only a small number of people in

England a rise in health consultations due to infection was noted, with 40 per cent of people consulting a health professional each year. National crises over the emergence of BSE and CJD, meningitis outbreaks and the constant pressure by the NHS to cope with outbreaks of winter influenza and bronchitis have also been problematic.

Alongside these changing infection rates, a new and emerging threat from war and terrorism has prompted health professionals and government officials to rethink their infections strategies. The attack on the Twin Towers and Washington DC on 11 September 2001 also served to reinforce the need to be diligent with the potential for disease as a result of such terrorist actions. Also, with the increases in world travel and as a result of the ease with which we can now cross continents, the emergence of disease in other parts of the world has caused some public concern.

As mentioned in Chapter 2 the influenza pandemic in 1918–19 killed 25 million people and the growing number of strains of the virus has caused experts to remark that it is not a question of whether such an outbreak will occur again but when. Already we have witnessed the emergence of so called 'bird flu', which was first found in chickens in Hong Kong. The first human case in 1991 led to some alarm but the outbreaks were stopped by the cull of 400 000 birds and 1.2 million chickens. However, more recently, the strain H5N1 has emerged in chickens in Britain and, alarmingly, this is the type that can be transmitted to humans.

The Health Protection Agency (HPA)

So, how can we deal with the rising tide of infection that threatens our economy, our security and our lives? The action proposed was to create a new National Infection Control and Health Protection Agency to replace the Public Health Laboratory Service, the National Radiological Protection Board, the Centre for Applied Microbiology and Research and the National Focus for Chemical Incidents. This new agency is the Health Protection Agency (**www.hpa.org.uk**) whose role is to provide an 'integrated approach to protecting UK public health through the provision of support and advice to the NHS, local authorities, emergency services, other Arm's Length Bodies, the Department of Health and the Devolved Administrations' (DoH, 2005).

The Health Protection Agency was established as a special health authority (SpHA) in 2003 and came in to being in 2004 when the relevant Act of Parliament was passed. It has the following functions:

a) the protection of the community (or any part of the community) against infectious diseases and other dangers to health;

b) the prevention and spread of infectious disease;

c) the provision of assistance to any other person who exercises functions in relation to the matters mentioned in paragraphs (a) and (b).

(**www.opsi.gov.uk/ACTS/acts2004/40017–a.htm**)

The HPA is:

- a local health protection service working with the NHS to deliver preventative, investigatory and control functions for infectious diseases;
- a national expert panel to assess threat;
- a surveillance system with an up-to-date data capture system which will integrate information from human infections with that from animals and the environment;
- a provider of action plans to address infectious disease priorities;
- a rationalisation of microbiology laboratories and the introduction of standards;
- an inspector of microbiology to ensure standards are being met;
- a programme of vaccine development;
- a source of better public information;
- a new research programme and a review of the law on infection control.

So, a new regime for the control of infection had been born and action plans have been put in place to fight the ever-increasing risk to our economy and the nation's health.

Winning Ways

In December 2003 the DoH report *Winning Ways: Working Together to Reduce Healthcare Associated Infection in England* was published and commented largely upon the state of affairs with respect to infections in hospitals (DoH, 2003c). Several initiatives have been put into place to reduce infections and included the following:

- checklists and control assurance standards to ensure the management of the environment to minimise infection risk;
- a mandatory surveillance scheme for serious bloodstream infections including MRSA, started in 2001;
- guidelines produced by NICE in 2003 on the prevention of health care infections in the community and primary care settings;
- the incorporation of two new performance management indicators related to infection control in the star ratings systems for hospitals (2003);
- the introduction of *Essential Steps to Safe, Clean Care* (DoH, 2006d).

Despite these guidelines and the vast drive to improve the situation in the health care setting it was apparent from this report that the degree of improvement had been small since their publication. Analysis of trends in surgical site infection showed that while there had been a degree of improvement in some hospitals (a 12 per cent reduction in infection), the majority of hospitals had shown no improvement at all and 2.5 per cent of hospitals had increased infection rates.

The publication in this paper of the then current position with respect to the health care risks highlighted the following points:

- Infection is common and sometimes life threatening.
- An examination of the world wide infection problem reveals the NHS in England as underperforming when compared with other European countries.
- The application of countermeasures being employed in hospitals is not consistent.
- Antibiotic resistance is on the increase making infection very hard to treat.
- The strains of MRSA, VRE and penicillin-resistant *Streptococcus pneumoniae* indicate high risk to some patients.

One of the major areas of concern had been the emergence of news that health care staff were failing in their basic duties to patients with respect to hand washing and, moreover, this was thought to be due to laziness or carelessness. Other barriers to hand hygiene also emerged. A lack of knowledge and education on the part of the health care worker about hygiene guidelines was one factor but the inadequate facilities and lack of time were also identified as part of the problem.

The EPIC Initiative

The emergence of the EPIC Guidelines (**www.epic.tvu.ac.uk**) in 1998 was the result of a series of long-term government-commissioned research projects that had as their main focus the development of the evidence base underpinning the practice of infection prevention and control in the NHS. In collaboration with the Infection Prevention Society (IPS), the Hospital Infection Society (HIS) and the Health Protection Agency (HPA) the guidelines were largely funded by the Department of Health and are currently available to view on the website given above. Various phased initiatives are in place as shown below.

- **EPIC phase 1** – Developing national evidence-based guidelines for preventing health care associated infections in NHS Hospitals 1999–2001. (These guidelines address the standard principles in the prevention of infection and give specific recommendations in relation to the use of short-term indwelling urethral catheters and central venous catheters.)

- **EPIC Phase 1a** – Supporting NHS Trusts to implement national guidance for preventing health care associated infections 2003–2005.
- **EPIC Phase 1b** – Updating the Phase 1 Guidelines 2004–2005.
- **EPIC Phase 2a** – Developing national evidence-based guidelines for preventing HAI in primary and community care services 2001–2003.
- **EPIC Phase 2a** – Infection control: prevention of health care associated infection in primary and community care. (These guidelines focus on primary and community care and were developed under the auspices of NICE.)
- **EPIC Phase 2b** – A National Review of the Role and Responsibilities of Community Infection Control Nurses (CICN) and Communicable Disease Control Nurses (CDCN) in England 2001–2002.
- **EPIC Phase 3** – Enhancing the Evidence-base for Infection Prevention and Control Practices in the United Kingdom (CHART) 2003–2006.
- **EPIC international** – A comparison of international practices in the management and control of health care association infections 2003–2004.
- **EPIC MRSA evidence review** – Systematic review of interventions to prevent the transmission of meticillin-resistant *Staphylococcus aureus* (MRSA) in hospitals 2004–2005.
- **EPIC 2** – Updated National Evidence-Based Guidelines for Preventing Healthcare-Associated Infections in NHS Hospitals in England.

These much used and quoted guidelines have provided an excellent information source and knowledge base for the furtherance of infection control in hospitals in order to reduce the ever-rising infection rates.

Activity 5

Visit the website **www.epic.tvu.ac.uk** and click on 'Phase 3 -- Enhancing the Evidence-base for Infection Prevention and Control Practices in the United Kingdom (CHART) 2003--2006'. Then go to the search box at the top of the page and check out the many related sites you can access to help you with your infection control work. Make a list of these websites.

Essential Steps to Safe, Clean Care

A further initiative which developed as a result of all the ongoing work and research into the reduction of health care associated infections was

Essential Steps to Safe, Clean Care: Reducing Healthcare-Associated Infections (DoH, 2006d). This project is the outcome of a collaboration with and research by the NHS Institute for Innovation and Improvement to adapt the *Saving Lives* delivery programme for community and non-acute settings.

Activity 6

Download a copy of the *Essential Steps* pack now from **www.clean-safe-care.nhs.uk**.

The pack aims to promote best practice to prevent and manage the spread of infections and ultimately improve patient and service user safety. The pack contains the following:

- signposting to useful information for users;
- three key essential steps that may impact significantly on reducing the level of infections;
- review tools to monitor compliance and to record continuous compliance or improvement in all work settings;
- certificates for staff to recognise their progress in performing safer practice;
- posters to provide simple safety messages to both staff and visitors.

The Essential Skills Clusters

The Essential Skills Clusters **www.nmc-uk.org/aFrameDisplay.aspx?DocumentID=3663** (2007) have been developed by the Nursing and Midwifery Council (2007) to ensure that all registered nurses are competently dealing with effective infection control. The Essential Skills Clusters were fully integrated in nurse training programmes in 2008 and identify the necessary skills required to practise as a nurse in this country.

Deep cleaning

Finally, the Prime Minister Gordon Brown recently pledged to rid the health service of fatal superbugs like MRSA in the *Observer* on 23 September 2007. He stated that every hospital in Britain was to undergo a ward-by-ward 'deep clean' within the next year to rid them of fatal superbugs such as MRSA. He said that 'walls, ceilings and ventilation shafts in hospitals across the country would be scrubbed clean'. The initiative is based on the experience from the USA, where 'deep cleans' are regularly carried out. NHS Trusts decide how to carry out the cleaning, with some wards being closed for a week at a time.

SUMMARY

It is clear that the problem of controlling infection within our health care settings has been a major issue for government for years. The White Paper entitled *A First Class Service: Quality in the New NHS* (DoH, 1998) outlined the principles of clinical governance and the initiative to put clinical quality at the heart of all NHS and community services business. It led to the development and setting up of various initiatives to try to control the rising tide of infection.

In terms of the legal aspects of health care we have covered the following legislation in this chapter. The Health and Safety at Work Act 1974 covers a range of legislation relating to the work environment and highlights the responsibility of the employer and employee with respect to safe standards of practice. The Public Health (Infectious Diseases) Regulations 1988 detail the need to notify infections to a central board and report incidences with respect to disease. New controls on hazardous waste came into force in England, Wales and Northern Ireland on 16 July 2005 replacing the previous 'Special Waste Regime'.

The DoH publication in 2002 *Getting Ahead of the Curve: A Strategy for Combating Infectious Diseases (Including Other Aspects of Health Protections)* and the government's White Paper *Saving Lives: A Delivery Programme to Reduce Healthcare-Associated Infection Including MRSA* (DoH, 2005) and led to a raft of initiatives to address the issues it outlined.

The emergence of the EPIC Guidelines in 1998 was the result of a series of long-term government-commissioned research projects that had as their main focus the development of the evidence base underpinning the practice of infection prevention and control in the NHS. The development of *Essential Steps to Safe, Clean Care: Reducing Healthcare-Associated Infections* (2006d) is the outcome of a collaboration with and research by the NHS Institute for Innovation and Improvement to adapt the *Saving Lives* delivery programme to community and non-acute settings.

We continue with the battle against infection and in Chapter 4 we will develop our understanding about cleaning and waste management.

Summary Activity

In order to fulfil the key learning outcomes for the Skills for Care Knowledge Set complete the following activity.

Within this chapter we have covered the key legislation, policies, documents, etc. that have had the most impact on infection control. These include:

- The Health and Safety at Work Act 1974
- The NICE Guidelines
- The Health Protection Agency
- The Hazardous Waste Regulations

1. Check that you understand the legislation, regulations and guidance that govern infection prevention and control by writing short notes on the legislation that is appropriate for your own care setting.

2. Ensure that you have a clear understanding of your organisation's policies and procedures with regard to infection prevention and control by preparing a checklist for new staff which summarises the policy.

Answers to the activities

Activity 5

Below are some websites that will provide you with useful information on infection prevention and control:

- The Richard Wells Research Centre at Thames Valley University: **www.richardwellsresearch.com/richardwells**
- The Health Protection Agency (UK): **www.hpa.org.uk**
- Centers for Disease Control and Prevention (USA): **www.cdc.gov**
- DHQP (Division of Healthcare Quality Promotion) (USA) (formerly HICPAC): **www.cdc.gov/ncidod/dhqp**
- Hospital Infection Society (UK): **www.his.org.uk**
- Infection Prevention Society (UK): **www.ips.uk.net**
- Infectious Diseases Society of America: **www.idsociety.org**
- APIC (Association for Professionals in Infection Control and Epidemiology, Inc.) (USA): **www.apic.org//AM/Template.cfm?Section=Home1**
- Health Canada Division of Nosocomial and Occupational Infections: **www.phac-aspc.gc.ca/publicat/ccdr-rmtc/02vol28/28s1/index.html**
- National Foundation for Infectious Diseases (USA): **www.nfid.org**

- Community and Hospital Infection Control Association (Canada): **www.chica.org**

Notes to help with the Summary Activity

The Health and Safety at Work Act 1974:

- an umbrella act;
- relates to work environment and highlights the responsibility of the employer and employee with respect to safety at work;
- statutory responsibilities to maintain safety at work, provide equipment and clothing if necessary for the job, ensure training is undertaken and provide a policy for working safely;
- employees must co-operate with policy and employer.

NICE Guidelines – NICE was set up in 1999 to:

- appraise practices in the NHS;
- produce clinical guidelines;
- introduce and develop audit procedures and confidential enquiries.

Health Protection Agency:

- replaced the Public Health Laboratory service;
- protects the public through providing support and advice to local authorities;
- known as a special health authority;
- set up to prevent and protect against spread of disease;
- set up to provide assistance to all people involved in health care.

Hazardous Waste Regulations:

- new guidelines introduced in 2005;
- notification must be made to the Environment Agency of any waste that is likely to be a hazard to health.

Chapter 4

Cleaning and Waste Management

In this chapter you will cover the following standards:

- Skills for Care Knowledge Set on Infection Prevention and Control
  2. Preventing and controlling the spread of infection
     2.1 Understand the standard precautions to prevent infection and its spread
     2.2 Understand the correct procedures for handling, storage and disposal of waste (using the correct colour-coded bag or bin)
     2.3 Understand decontamination techniques
- Skills for Health Infection Prevention and Control Competencies:
  IPC1, IPC3, IPC4, IPC8, IPC9, IPC10, IPC11, IPC12

See also:
RCN (2005a) *Good Practice in Infection Prevention and Control –* Section 4: Understand the standard precautions to prevent infection and its spread.

INTRODUCTION

In Chapter 3 we discussed briefly the advent of Standard Universal Precautions and in this chapter we will develop your understanding of these important guidelines.

Activity 1

Using a blank sheet of paper create a mind map of what you can recall about the Standard Universal Precautions we discussed in Chapter 3.

An example of a mind map and answers to all relevant activities are given at the end of the chapter.

You may have recalled some of the following points:

- The Standard Universal Precautions were developed by the Centers for Disease Control in 1985.

- The Advisory Committee on Dangerous Pathogens issued guidelines that were to be applied in all nursing and medical procedures.
- The Standard Universal Precautions are a set of precautions or broad principles that are designed to prevent the transmission of human immunodeficiency virus (HIV), hepatitis B virus (HBV) and other blood-borne pathogens when providing any form of health or medical care.
- It is imperative that care workers consider all patients to be a source of infection.
- Infections such as those caused by droplet or airborne means, influenza and tuberculosis, still require isolation nursing techniques to be in place and we will come back to this later in the chapter.
- In the USA, the system of Body Substance Isolation (BSI) has been introduced but the Standard Precautions are incorporated into the general guidelines.
- Standard Universal Precautions apply to blood and any bodily fluid containing visible blood.

Let's now look more closely at how these guidelines can be incorporated into our practice to prevent the spread of infection. As we have seen, Standard Universal Precautions refer to

> the set of precautions or broad principles which are designed to prevent transmission of human immunodeficiency virus (HIV), hepatitis B virus (HBV), and other blood-borne pathogens when providing any form of health or medical care.
> **(www.cdc.gov/ncidod/dhqp/bp_universal_precautions.html)**

These precautions are fine if the patient presents with an infection and procedures are put into place to isolate that infection. But what of the conditions that are infectious before any signs appear? The patient with MRSA is often asymptomatic and the child with chicken pox is infectious before the spots appear. In these cases cross infection is likely to occur and puts patients and health care workers at risk. It is therefore imperative for all care workers to use infection controls as a routine measure for all patients regardless of known infections. All patients are therefore viewed as potentially infectious and in the late 1980s it was recommended that practices be adopted to reduce the risk of cross contamination.

The Centers for Disease Control in Atlanta in 1985 recommended the use of Standard Universal Precautions, recognised that these practices, if adopted by care workers, would minimise the risk of cross infection greatly. The core principles of infection control were proposed to be:

- effective hand washing and hygiene;
- protective clothing and equipment;

- isolation nursing;
- laundry management;
- waste management;
- cleanliness of the environment;
- decontamination of equipment;
- management of bodily fluids and exposure to blood.

We shall deal with each of these in turn.

EFFECTIVE HAND WASHING AND HYGIENE

With such a wealth of hand hygiene studies at our disposal there is still a lot of evidence to suggest that compliance may still be a problem. In other words, we all know that we need to wash our hands but we don't necessarily do it or, if we do it, we do it ineffectively.

Dirty hands are the most common way in which infection can be spread, and we have known about the importance of good hand hygiene for more than a hundred years. Medical advice for doctors to wash their hands came as a result of the mid-nineteenth-century work by obstetrician and infection control pioneer Ignaz Semmelweis of the Vienna Lying-in Hospital in Austria. This advice prevented the deaths of many babies and their mothers. He noted that in one ward the deaths from childbed fever were significantly higher than in another ward. The only difference was in the personnel and the work they were doing prior to delivering babies. On the ward where the infection rate was high, Semmelweis observed that medical students were going straight from performing post mortems to delivering babies. On the other ward midwife students were practising and were therefore free from other duties where contamination might be a problem. Following the death of a colleague, who had cut himself while performing a post mortem and subsequently died from a condition similar to those who had childbed fever, Semmelweis was convinced of his claims. His reaction was to order the washing of hands before every delivery and this action brought about a dramatic reduction in deaths from childbed fever from 11 per cent to below 1 per cent.

Florence Nightingale also pointed to the need for

> Every nurse to be careful to wash her hands very frequently during the day. If her face too, so much the better.
>
> (Nightingale, 1860)

As you learned in Chapter 1 you are a walking host for pathogens and carry with you millions of microbes. Your hands are populated with micro-organisms which are acquired throughout your day and during the procedures you carry out. When an area you touch is moist or heavily contaminated with bacteria it is possible for the micro-organisms to survive long enough on your skin for them to be passed onto another person. Activities that have shown care workers acquiring pathogenic (disease causing) micro-organisms include:

- touching, lifting and washing a patient;
- changing babies' nappies;
- bed making and handling curtains;
- dressing a wound;
- respiratory care.

You also have micro-organisms on your skin that are there all the time and which live under your nails and in the deep crevices of your skin.

The majority of these microbes are removed with efficient hand washing but you will also be aware that studies have shown that there are certain parts of the hand that are frequently missed and will therefore still harbour microbes. Taylor (1978) observed nurses washing their hands and reported they were missing large areas of the hand. These areas were particularly the thumbs and fingertips. McGinley *et al.* (1988) carried out research on the existence of microbes in the subungual (beneath a nail) area of the hand. The findings supported the fact that nurses with long nails harboured more microbes and were therefore capable of transmitting infection to patients via this route (Moolenaar *et al.*, 2000).

So it is vital to reduce the risk by ensuring that all care professionals follow the principles outlined below:

- keep nails short;
- remove nail varnish and false nails before working with patients/clients;
- do not wear rings with stones or engravings;
- if you are wearing a wedding ring this must be moved during hand hygiene to facilitate soap and water or alcohol gel access to the area beneath the ring, and attention must be paid to drying the area beneath the ring as warm moist environments harbour micro-organisms;
- remove wristwatches before giving clinical care and during hand hygiene.

Another area which has come under scrutiny is the availability of hand washing facilities. In 2003 Sir Liam Donaldson made the following comment:

Common sense tells us that the cleanliness of our hospitals plays a part in infection control. We need to look at how infections move from person to person. Do staff, for example, have easily accessible facilities to disinfect their hands?

(Cited in **www.flemingforum.org.uk/slides/handwashing.pdf**)

It became apparent that one of the reasons why hand washing was not being carried out effectively was the lack of facilities to do so. This has led to the wider use of alcohol gel washes and hand rubs and, while not to be used as a complete substitute for soap and water, they do have their part to play in some settings. In many health and social care settings the use of alcohol gels and rubs has been made readily available, particularly on the entrance to wards in hospitals or at patient's bedsides. In other settings, this may be more problematic. It is the responsibility of all care workers to carry out hand decontamination before every care activity (EPIC Project 2001) and, in order to do this, care workers in community settings and working in clients' homes may need to carry their own liquid soap and paper towels. In some clients' homes hot and cold water and soap are readily available but, where this is an issue, then an alcohol hand hygiene rub may be used. We need to remember, however, that the use of an alcohol rub is not a substitute for removing dirt and washing frequently with soap and water is recommended.

For care homes the Department of Health document *Infection Control Guidance for Care Homes* (2006a) outlines the steps to prevent infection in this type of setting. If you are working in a care home you are advised to familiarise yourself with the document (see **www.dh.gov.uk/en/ Publicationsandstatistics/Publications/PublicationsPolicyAndGuidance /DH_4136381**).

Correct hand wash technique

Figure 1 shows the guidance from the WHO showing how the hands need to be washed to ensure that effective removal of microbes is achieved. The drawings have been adapted from the wide range of posters we now see in all areas of public life. Even public conveniences now display such information! You can download the *Essential Steps to Safe, Clean Care* pack which contains this particular work and gives more detail regarding the technique (see Chapter 3).

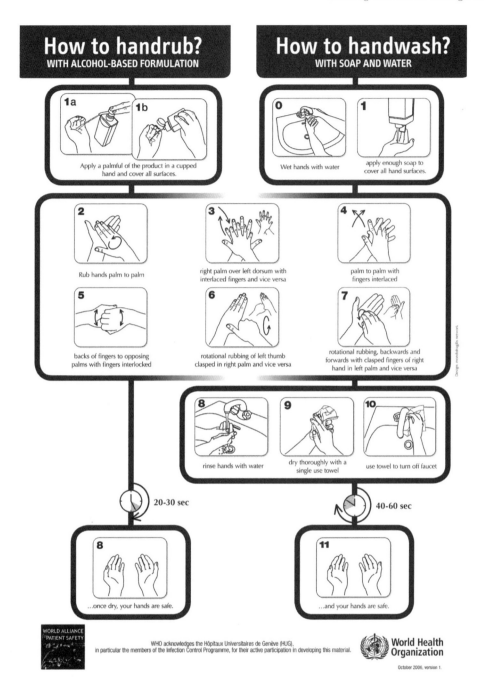

Figure 1 Hand washing and using hand rubs
Reproduced with permission from the World Health Organization.

The Ayliffe technique

Ayliffe *et al.* (1978) devised a six-step technique that is used to ensure that all parts of the hands are washed. This is shown in the WHO guidelines in Figure 1 and explained further below:

- **Step one** – under running water and using soap clean the hands by washing palms.
- **Step two** – right palm over left dorsum (the back of hand) and left palm over right dorsum.
- **Step three** – palm to palm with interlacing of fingers.
- **Step four** – backs of fingers to palms with fingers interlocked.
- **Step five** – rotational rubbing of each thumb in palms.
- **Step six** – rotational rubbing with clasped fingers of right hand in left palm and vice versa.

Following this rather prescriptive but most effective technique you need to be sure to rinse hands thoroughly and then dry them well, remembering that bacteria thrive in the warm and moist areas of our skin. It is imperative to use paper towels to dry your hands rather than a towel or roller towel that may be harbouring bacteria.

We are washing our hands constantly in the care setting and this can lead to chapping and soreness. In order to keep hands in good condition we need to take care of our hands at all times to maintain supple skin free from abrasions and cuts. A barrier cream may be effective to prevent dirt getting into the pores of the skin and should be applied with particular attention to the cuticles and underneath the fingernails. A moisturiser may be used as required to maintain skin suppleness. However, communal jars of hand cream can harbour bacteria so it is best to have hand cream in a pump dispenser.

Activity 2

Carry out an assessment of the hand washing facilities and procedures used in your care setting. Armed with the knowledge you now have of the correct procedure, is there any room for improvements to be made in your own care setting to improve this part of the infection control procedures?

PERSONAL PROTECTIVE CLOTHING AND EQUIPMENT

The purpose of any personal protective equipment (PPE) and clothing in the care setting is to prevent harmful pathogens from being transmitted via clothing to patients and staff. Under the Health and Safety at Work Act 1974 all employers have a duty to provide such clothing and, following a risk assessment in the clinical setting, employers will determine what PPE is required.

In areas where there is a high risk of contamination with blood and other bodily fluids there is likely to be a need for gloves, aprons, gowns and goggles as well as masks. In theatre areas of hospitals, for example, the risk of infection means that staff must use all precautions and protective clothing to prevent such occurrences. In a care home it is likely you will only require gloves and aprons as the risk of infection is less severe.

Activity 3

Carry out a risk assessment in your own work setting. What protective clothing do you think you require and why?

Inform your manager of the outcome of your findings.

Gloves

Gloves should be worn:

- for touching blood and body fluids, mucous membranes or non-intact skin of all patients; and
- for handling items or surfaces soiled with blood or body fluids.

Gloves should be changed after contact with each client and hands and other skin surfaces should be washed immediately or as soon as possible. Remember that:

- gloves should only be used once and must never be washed;
- gloves must be discarded following the correct procedure;
- gloves must conform to European Union standards.

The type of glove needed depends upon the procedure for which it is being used. In all surgery a sterile glove must be available and can be latex or a synthetic alternative. For examination purposes latex or synthetic alternatives are available and are either sterile or non-sterile. A good rule of thumb to employ is that all procedures where asepsis is required (for example, catheter insertion and dressing changes) a sterile glove needs to be employed. For other purposes where there is a risk of exposure to blood or bodily fluids non-sterile gloves can be used.

Aprons

Gowns or aprons should be worn during procedures that are likely to generate splashes of blood or body fluids. Remember that:

- aprons are for single use only;
- they should be discarded following use;
- they should be stored in a clean dry area away from sources of contamination.

Masks and goggles

Outside of the theatre environment masks are not routinely used. However, where there might be the potential for blood splashes (for example, in dentistry) or if there is a suspected TB infection then masks should be used.

Uniforms

Studies by Perry *et al.* (2001) and Babb (1983) have shown that uniforms are a potential source of contamination from *Staphylococcus aureus* and *Clostridium difficile* and, as such, staff need to be diligent in ensuring that they are changed daily and are not worn outside. Staff should change out of their uniforms before they go home from work and should wash their uniforms at 65°C and dry them thoroughly.

The RCN has produced guidelines to ensure that all staff are aware of the need to adhere to such infection control measures with respect to uniforms. The guidance can be found in the RCN *Wipe it Out* campaign on MRSA (see **www.rcn.org.uk/search?queries_seach_query=wipe+it +out**).

ISOLATION NURSING

Isolation or 'barrier' nursing is a term used to denote the separation of a client or patient with an infective disorder from others to prevent the spread of the condition. It is by no means a new concept as it has been used for over one hundred years when caring for patients known or thought to be suffering from a contagious disease such as tuberculosis. In the early twentieth century these patients were often nursed in the so called 'fever hospitals', thus separating them entirely from patients with other conditions. This was felt to be a more useful way of dealing with infections that were airborne in nature as it was impossible to isolate these patients in the old type of Nightingale Wards where rows of beds afforded little opportunity to 'isolate' a condition. The newer types of hospitals with their smaller bays of four beds and single occupancy rooms have made isolation and barrier nursing easier.

All contagious patients are isolated in separate rooms but, if this is not possible and the condition is not of the airborne transmission variety, then the patient is nursed in a ward with others with screens placed around the bed. This is sometimes termed 'bed isolation'.

Care workers are instructed to wear gowns, masks and gloves, and they observe strict rules to minimise the risk of passing on infectious agents. This includes the following protocols.

All equipment and utensils used to care for the patient are immediately placed in a bowl of sterilising solution. Crockery can be removed to the kitchen for the usual cleaning.

- Nurses and care workers observe surgical standards of cleanliness in hand washing after they have been attending the patient.
- Bedding is carefully moved in order to minimise the transmission of airborne particles, such as dust or droplets, which could carry contagious material.
- Bedding is bagged and removed for special cleaning that includes the use of steam heat for sterilisation.
- Visitors must observe all of the above precautions.

Activity 4

If you work in a health care organisation, obtain a copy of your Isolation or Barrier Nursing policy. Does it clearly state the following?

1. An indication of when the isolation policy is invoked.
2. The aims of the policy.
3. The equipment made available to the client e.g. bedpans.
4. The procedure regarding PPE, hand washing, disposal of waste and linen, visitors and cleaning procedures.
5. The reasons for the procedures.

If there is no such policy use the guidelines above to write your own.

THE HANDLING, STORAGE AND DISPOSAL OF WASTE

In all health and social care settings you can expect to generate waste such as towels, dressings, needles and syringes, as well as linen and bodily waste. The Environmental Protection Act 1990 outlines the responsibilities of those who produce waste and give guidance on the correct and safe methods of disposal.

Most of the waste we produce in health care settings is termed 'clinical waste' and, as such, it is subject to stringent methods of disposal. Clinical waste is defined by the Controlled Waste Regulations 1992 as any waste that consists wholly or partly of:

- blood or other bodily fluids;
- drugs or other pharmaceutical products;
- excretions;
- human or animal tissue;
- swabs or dressings;
- syringes, needles or other sharp instruments which may be hazardous to anybody who comes in contact with them.

It is also useful for you to be aware of the following main pieces of legislation:

- Environmental Protection Act 1990: **www.opsi.gov.uk/acts/acts1990/ Ukpga_19900043_en_1.htm**;
- Special Waste Regulations 1996 (SI 1996/942) (some clinical waste is also classified as special waste and the Environment Agency has issued technical guidance on the definition);
- Waste Management Licensing Regulations 1994 (SI 1994/1056);
- Environmental Protection (Duty of Care) Regulations 1991 (SI 1991/ 2839): **www.envirowise.gov.uk/ref028**

The Health Services Advisory Committee's (1999) guidance document *Safe Disposal of Clinical Waste* has now been updated by the Health Technical Memorandum 07-01 (DoH, 2006b) to take into account the changes in legislation governing the management of waste, its storage, carriage, treatment and disposal, and health and safety. Carry out the task in the next activity to ensure you have a good idea of where the information for safe handling of clinical waste can be obtained.

Activity 5

Visit the website **www.dh.gov.uk** and type in the following text in the 'search' box at the top of the page:

Health Technical Memorandum 07-01: Safe Management of Healthcare Waste.

This 120-page document has been produced as a best practice guide to the management of health care waste.

You do not need to download or print the whole document unless you feel it would be needed in your work setting. Just dip into it and familiarise yourself with the guidance given. Look in particular at section 7 which deals with waste segregation and the national colour-coding system.

Hazardous and non-hazardous waste

Since July 2005 new regulations from the Environment Agency have made it necessary to classify waste from clinical areas in to 'hazardous' and 'non-hazardous' types. Hazardous waste refers to material that is potentially toxic and may therefore cause disease. You are required to dispose of hazardous waste by incineration.

So why is it so important that we cover hazardous waste in this book? The Audit Commission has published figures that state that the NHS generates 193 000 tonnes of clinical waste every year (Audit Commission 1997) with acute wards producing an average of 0.2 tonnes of waste per bed per week.

There has also been an increase in the amount of clinical waste coming from households. Self-injecting diabetics and people changing colostomy bags at home can also generate significant quantities of clinical waste. With early discharge from hospital it is also possible that dressings will require changing at home thus producing more waste. Clinical waste represents a risk both to people and to the environment if it is not handled correctly and it accounts for two primary risks – infection and toxicity.

In Table 1 (page 82) you will note the various categories of waste and the way they are to be disposed of (DoH, 2006b).

Have you thought about the way in which your own care setting disposes of waste and the costs involved in this disposal? If you put all the waste into yellow bags the cost of disposal is more than double that of the cost of waste in black bags. In 1997 the Audit Commission produced a report confirming the problem associated with the lack of waste segregation in the health service. General waste is frequently disposed of in clinical waste receptacles (for example, in yellow bags) and the cost of clinical waste disposal is between £180–£320 per tonne. This is up to nine times more than the figure for household waste, which is between £20–£70 per tonne (Audit Commission, 1997). Therefore, by implementing the following measures, you may actually find the cost of your own care setting's waste disposal could be radically reduced:

Group	Description of type of waste	Colour of disposal container	Method of disposal
A	Includes the following items: identifiable human tissue, blood, animal carcasses and the tissue from veterinary centres, hospitals or laboratories. Soiled surgical dressings, swabs and all other similar soiled waste. Any infectious waste material excluded from Groups B–E	Yellow or light blue or transparent with blue lettering.	This should be disposed of by incineration.
B	Discarded syringes, needles, cartridges, broken glass and other contaminated disposable sharp instruments or items.	Yellow sharps boxes.	
C	Microbiological cultures and potentially infected waste from pathology departments and other clinical or research laboratories.	Yellow or orange depending upon the type of waste.	Some waste may require incineration or just treatment.
D	Drugs or other pharmaceutical products.	Yellow.	For incineration.
E	Items used to dispose of urine, faeces and other bodily secretions and excretions that do not fall within Group A. This includes used disposable bedpans or bedpan liners, incontinence pads, stoma bags, catheter bags and tubes and urine containers.	Yellow with black stripe.	Non-infectious waste, e.g. Group E and sanitary products, which is suitable for landfill or other means of disposal.
	Non-clinical and household waste.	Black.	

Table 1 Categories of waste and method of disposal

- the training of relevant staff – doctors and cleaners were found to be poorly trained in clinical waste management;
- clear signs and instructions for staff;
- an ample supply of coded waste sacks;
- a system of communication with staff over the need for and implications of a good waste segregation policy (Ison, 1998).

While on the subject of disposing waste, one time at which we are at risk during such procedures is when we are disposing of equipment such as needles and syringes. We will cover this more fully in Chapter 5 but, briefly, the following should be taken into consideration:

- To prevent needlestick injuries, needles should not be recapped, or bent or broken by hand, removed from disposable syringes, or otherwise manipulated by hand.
- After use, disposable syringes and needles, scalpel blades and other sharp items should be placed in puncture-resistant containers for disposal (yellow bins with instructions written on the sides in red and black).
- The puncture-resistant containers should be located as close to the use area as possible.
- All reusable needles should be placed in a puncture-resistant container for transport to the reprocessing area.

In Chapter 5 we will look at what to do should you or any of your colleagues sustain a needlestick injury.

Future trends in waste management

The regulations for the management of clinical waste are currently being changed. Clinical waste which is classified as special waste will be subject to the requirements of the EU Landfill Directive 99/31 (see **www.waste online.org.uk/resources/Wasteguide/mn_legislation_european_euaffect. html**) and pre-treatment will be required for all such clinical wastes prior to landfill. Hospital, infectious clinical waste and waste drugs will be banned from landfill and will require special decontamination processes to be carried out before being sent to special sites.

UNDERSTANDING DECONTAMINATION TECHNIQUES

Decontamination refers to the ways in which we can render an environment clean and free from the possible risks of infection. There are three types of decontamination:

1. cleaning;
2. disinfection;
3. sterilisation.

In selecting one of the above methods we need to be very clear about the infection risk relating to the use of the item to be cleaned. Have a look at the following activity and determine how you might decontaminate the equipment listed.

Activity 6

For each of the following items, identify whether the method of decontamination is cleaning, disinfection or sterilisation.

- bedpans
- peak flow meters
- stethoscope
- vaginal speculum
- urinals
- nailbrushes
- thermometers

- bowls
- beds
- surgical instruments
- razors
- laryngoscope blades
- mattresses
- catheters

Your choice of method will depend upon the risk of infection associated with each of the items listed above. In fact, you needed to carry out a risk assessment and your own local policy for decontamination should specify the protocols you should use in your area. Guidance on the decontamination of equipment was provided by the Medical Devices Agency (1996). The risks are classified as shown in Table 2.

Level of risk	Indication	Examples	Contamination level	Methods of decontamination
High	In close contact with a break in the skin or mucous membrane. Introduced into sterile body area.	Surgical instruments. Needles and syringes. Catheters.	Sterilise	Using an autoclave and/or single-use items that can be disposed of following use.
Intermediate	In contact with mucous membranes. Contaminated with virulent or transmissible organisms prior to use on immuno-compromised patients.	Vaginal speculum. Bedpans, cutlery and crockery. Razors. Thermometers.	Disinfect or sterilise	Use of chemical disinfections or autoclave.
Low	Any item used on intact skin.	Washbowls, mattresses, beds.	Clean	Wash with detergent and dry thoroughly.

Table 2 Classification of risk and decontamination

Cleaning

Water and detergent are the best way to remove surface dirt and grease and to render the item free of a large number of micro-organisms. Cleaning should also be undertaken prior to disinfecting items and sterilising them. After cleaning it is very important that items are dried thoroughly. As we mentioned earlier, damp items are a good breeding ground for bacteria and, in a study by Greaves (1985), damp bowls were found to be harbouring **Gram negative** bacilli that are readily transferred to the next patient unlucky enough to be using the bowl.

The following list of cleaning equipment and methods have been suggested by the Medical Devices Agency.

Equipment

- A sink or a bowl that will hold a sufficient volume of water/detergent so that the item of equipment to be cleaned can be fully immersed.
- A warm, compatible water/detergent solution at the correct dilution and temperature, i.e. not greater than 35°C.
- Brush(es) and jet washer/handspray.
- A receptacle to contain rinse water such as, for example, a second sink and a drainage surface.
- A clean, disposable, absorbent, non-shedding cloth or mechanical drying facility like, for example, a drying cabinet or industrial hot air dryer.
- A chemical neutraliser, first aid kit and eye wash bottle in case of splashing with detergent.

(Adapted from the MDA Guidance 18 MAC
Manual Part 2 – Protocols, April 2005)

Cleaning procedure

- Ensure that the cleaning receptacle is clean and dry.
- Wearing protective clothing fill the sink or receptacle with sufficient warm water/detergent solution to ensure complete immersion of the item.
- Equipment should be dismantled where necessary, in line with the manufacturer's instructions, before cleaning.
- Carefully immerse the item in the solution in order to displace trapped air; it is important to ensure that the cleaning solution reaches all surfaces including the internal surfaces of lumened or cannulated devices.
- Brush, wipe, agitate, irrigate, jet wash or hand spray the item to dislodge and remove all visible soiling, taking care that the action is undertaken beneath the surface of the solution.
- Remove the item from the solution and drain over the detergent solution before transferring to a clean-rinse receptacle or sink.

- Rinse item thoroughly with clean water or with a water jet gun, ensuring that the item being rinsed is fully immersed.
- Remove item from rinse water and drain.
- Carefully hand-dry using absorbent, non-shedding cloth or industrial hot air dryer, or place into a drying cabinet.
- Thoroughly wash and dry items before storing and reuse.
- Used brushes should be decontaminated after use and discarded if there are signs of wear.

Some larger items cannot be immersed and therefore require a different method of cleaning. The MDA gives clear guidance as to how this is to be achieved.

Cleaning procedure for large items

- If the item is electrical, ensure that it is disconnected from the mains supply before commencing the cleaning procedure.
- Wearing protective clothing, immerse the cleaning cloth in the detergent solution and wring thoroughly.
- Commencing with the upper surface of the item, wipe thoroughly ensuring that the detergent solution does not enter electrical components.
- Periodically rinse the cloth in clean water and repeat the above steps.
- Surfaces should be carefully hand-dried using a cloth or industrial hot air dryer or placed into a drying cabinet.

Note that non-immersion, manual cleaning is not a disinfection process, but where an alcohol wipe is used to dry surfaces, this may have a disinfecting effect. Safely dispose of cleaning materials and alcohol wipes, if used.

Disinfection

This is achieved with the use of chemicals, either by immersion or in industrial chemical washers. Unfortunately, this method of decontamination carries risks to the care worker. Many of the chemicals used to achieve disinfection are skin irritants and special precautions need to be taken. It is vital that the most up-to-date version of the Control of Substances Hazardous to Health (COSHH) Regulations are followed here and the employer must ensure that risk assessments have been carried out on the use of the disinfectants to be used. Protective clothing will need to be worn and the correct dilution of the chemical to be used must be followed.

Common chemical disinfectants you may come across

Some of the more common chemical disinfectants you may come across are given in Table 3.

Type of disinfectant	Some brand names	Applications	Uses	Dilution
Alcohol	Ethanol, methylated spirit, alcohol impregnated wipes, alcohol handrubs.	Skin disinfections. Trolleys. Thermo-meters.	Effective on bacteria and some viruses. Good for skin disinfections and clean surfaces. It is flammable and can damage plastic and rubber.	Ethanol 70% (90% for viral disinfection).
Chlor-hexidine	Hibitane. Hibiscrub. Hibisol.	Used mainly for skin disinfection, particularly in theatres.	Gram positive/negative bacteria and fungi and some viruses.	1 in 10 (0.5%) with alcohol for pre-op. 1 in 100 (0.05%) for general skin disinfection.
Gluteralde-hyde	Glutaralde-hyde.	Formaldehyde.	Heat sensitive equipment and some surgical instruments. Not recommended for use outside of hospitals.	Kills bacteria, fungi, viruses in 20-60 minutes and spores in 3-10 hours. Can be used on heat-sensitive
equipment but is highly toxic and must therefore be	used cautiously.	Strictly controlled and not	recommended.	**Phenolics**
Jeyes Fluid, IZAL, Stercol, Clearsil and Hycolin.	Environmental disinfection.	Gram positive/negative bacteria and fungi and some viruses. They are irritants.	Tercol 1% Hycolin 1% Clearsil 0.625%. Others – follow instructions.	**Hypo-chlorites**

Table 3 Common chemical disinfectants

Disinfection requires items to be cleaned thoroughly before being immersed in disinfectant solution as the effectiveness of a disinfectant relies on good contact between the disinfectant and the item to be disinfected.

Disinfectants can cause irritation to the skin, eyes, mucous membranes and respiratory tract and can also be flammable and corrosive so the decision for use must be taken carefully. If an item can be washed thoroughly and it is not necessary to disinfect then this should suffice. Following disinfection all irritant disinfectant residues should be removed before the item is reused (adapted from the MDA Guidance 32 MAC Manual Part 2 – Protocols, April 2005).

Environmental disinfection

There has been much guidance of late about the use of disinfection to control infection in the clinical environment. The government's new 'Deep Clean' initiative will undoubtedly use some of the guidance we have looked at above in its methods. *The Code of Practice for the Prevention and Control of Healthcare Associated Infections* (DoH, 2006c) makes it clear to NHS bodies that they have a duty to provide and maintain a clean and appropriate environment. The Deep Clean Project is just one of a wide range of measures introduced by the government to tackle health care associated infections and ensure patient safety and confidence.

Activity 7

Check your own protocols for the cleaning arrangements in your care setting and determine what changes might need to be made.

Floors and walls

It goes without saying that the environment must be kept clean and dry to prevent the growth of micro-organisms and I expect you are familiar with the use of damp dusting as a means to achieve this. However, remember that cloths, mop heads and buckets all need to be cleaned thoroughly before and after use and stored away dry.

Toilet and bathroom areas

Being moist environments we would expect toilets and bathrooms to be potential areas for micro-organism growth. However, many studies have shown this to be unfounded. Regular cleaning with detergents is usually found to be effective and it is only in outbreaks of gastroenteritis that the use of disinfectants may be required.

The contamination found in baths and washbasins has been associated with the use of scourers when the surface of the bath becomes damaged and therefore a place where micro-organisms can thrive (Dowsett and Wilson, 1981).

Beds, cots and mattresses

It is not necessary to disinfect all mattresses and, provided they are clean, dry and the cover is intact, there should be no risk of transmission of bacteria to other patients. However, incubators do require the use of a hypochlorite solution to disinfect them between patients. Also, some humidification equipment may need disinfection and sterilising.

Sterilisation

Finally we look at decontamination by heat. This is the best method of decontaminating medical equipment and can be carried out using the following methods:

- pasteurisation;
- boiling;
- autoclaving;
- hot air ovens;
- irradiation.

Pasteurisation

This process, named after its creator Louis Pasteur, is the method of heating items for the purpose of destroying viruses, bacteria and other micro-organisms. The temperatures recommended are between 65 and 80°C, at which temperature many micro-organisms are destroyed. The items of equipment most likely to be treated in this way are those that present an intermediate risk in terms of infection transmission such as bedpans and linen. The optimum time for bedpans in a washer is at least one minute at 80°C and for bed linen 3 minutes at 71°C.

Boiling

Although not widely used it may have a place in the community setting to disinfect intermediate risk equipment. Most bacteria can be destroyed using this method but instruments must be immersed in boiling water for at least five minutes to clean them effectively.

Autoclaving

Water boiling in an enclosed space boils at a higher temperature because of the pressure created within the vessel. The steam that is produced will destroy micro-organisms and the higher the temperature the more spores will be destroyed. The definition supplied by **medicinenet.com** for an autoclave (see Figure 2) is:

> A chamber for sterilizing with steam under pressure. The original autoclave was essentially a pressure cooker. The steam tightened the lid. The device was called an autoclave (from the Greek *auto* 'self' and *clavis* 'key') meaning self-locking.

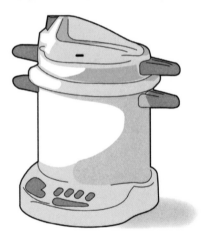

Figure 2 An autoclave

Autoclaves are the most common method of sterilising surgical instruments and keeping them sterile. Following the clinical procedure the instruments are placed in a sealed bag prior to being autoclaved. Intermediate risk equipment such as, for example, a speculum, which need not be retained sterile, can be stored in a clean environment following autoclaving.

Two types of autoclave may be used: vacuum-assisted or non-vacuum-assisted. Vacuum-assisted autoclaves are the most efficient at ensuring pre-packed instruments are sterilised and dried because steam has been allowed to penetrate all areas of the instrument due to the vacuum created inside the machine.

Non-vacuum-assisted autoclaves are simpler devices that are commonly used when instruments are not pre-packed and steam is allowed to condense on the surfaces of the instruments. They should therefore not be overloaded.

Hot air ovens

These are ovens that use a higher heat and longer time to ensure that articles are sterilised sufficiently.

Irradiation

This is mainly used in industry and is for the preparation of plastic items such as syringes.

Sterilisation can therefore be achieved by moist heat at raised pressure, by dry heat at normal pressure and by irradiation.

SUMMARY

If infection control is to become a well-managed part of your role as a professional care worker you need to fully understand the following:

- the standard precautions to prevent infection and its spread;
- the correct procedures for the handling, storage and disposal of waste (using the correct colour-coded bag or bins);
- decontamination techniques.

This chapter has set out the necessary guidance to equip you with this knowledge.

The chapter has also demonstrated the importance of hand hygiene as one of the most effective ways of ensuring that cross infection is minimised and has highlighted the importance of the use of protective equipment, not only for the patient/client but also for the care worker. Indeed, all employers have a duty to provide such clothing as required by the Health and Safety at Work Act 1974 and, in the clinical setting, a risk assessment will determine what is required.

With respect to the correct procedures for handling, storage and disposal of waste and decontamination techniques, the message is clear and protocols are outlined in the various government initiatives and legislation. *The Code of Practice for the Prevention and Control of Healthcare Associated Infections* states that NHS bodies have a duty to provide and maintain a clean and appropriate environment and the Deep Clean Project is just one of a wide range of measures introduced by the government to tackle health care associated infections and ensure patient safety and confidence. In all health and social care settings you can expect to generate waste in terms of towels, dressings, needles and syringes as well as linen and bodily waste. The Controlled Waste Regulations 1992 give guidance on how to ensure the correct procedures are followed in this respect.

The guidance in this chapter has been on the use of various strategies to minimise the infection rate and to control its spread. In the next chapter we will deal with the ways in which we can keep ourselves and our service users safe from the infections we are dealing with.

Answers to the activities

Activity 1

Figure 3 provides an example of a mind map regarding Standard Universal Precautions.

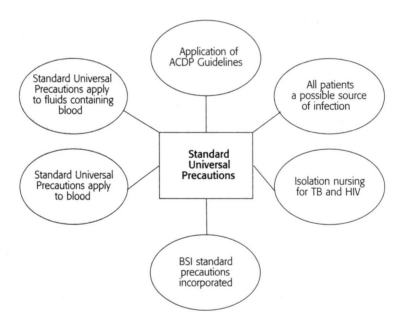

Figure 3 Example of a mind map

Activity 6

Method of decontamination:

- **bedpans** – if cardboard mash in machine and if metal then sterilise;
- **bowls** – clean and dry with disinfectant;
- **peak flow meters** – remove cardboard mouthpiece and discard then clean and disinfect;
- **beds** – clean and disinfect;
- **stethoscope** – clean and disinfect ear pieces and scope end;
- **surgical instruments** – clean and sterilise;
- **vaginal speculum** – clean and sterilise;
- **razors** – clean and disinfect or discard;
- **urinals** – clean and disinfect;
- **laryngoscope blades** – clean and disinfect (blades can be sterilised in liquid solution but cannot be autoclaved due to bulb);
- **mattresses** – clean and disinfect;
- **nailbrushes** – Should not be used now and need to be dispensed with. These are now only used in theatre settings;
- **thermometers** – clean and disinfect;
- **catheters** – discard or autoclave.

Chapter 5

Infection Control and Personal Hygiene – Keeping Yourself and Your Service Users Safe

---

In this chapter you will cover the following standards:

- Skills for Care Knowledge Set on Infection Prevention and Control
  4.3   Understand the need to carry out risk assessment when dealing with individuals and potentially contaminated materials.
- National Minimum Standards 11.2, 11.3, 11.4

See also:
- RCN (2005a) *Good Practice in Infection Prevention and Control* – Sections 1, 2, 5, 8 and 9.
- Department of Health (2006d) *Essential Steps to Safe, Clean Care*.
- EPIC Guidelines (Pratt *et al.*, 2001).

INTRODUCTION

Health care workers put themselves at risk of infection every time they set foot in the workplace and previous chapters have testified to this fact. We need therefore to address the responsibility we all have to keep ourselves free of infection and to protect ourselves and our service users in the workplace.

In Chapter 3 we started the process of assessing a risk in the workplace. In this chapter we shall take this a stage further and focus on the risks to our own and other people's health in the workplace with respect to infection and its prevention and control. We also looked briefly at the Health and Safety at Work Act 1974. Carry out the following activity to see what you can recall about that legislation.

Activity 1

Complete the following text by inserting the correct words. The words at the bottom of the activity will help and the answers to this and all relevant activities are given at the end of the chapter.

The Health and Safety at Work Act 1974 is known as an............(1) act covering a range of............(2) relating to the work environment and highlights the responsibility of the ....(3) and............(4) with respect to.............(5) standards of practice. All employers have a ....(6) responsibility to create a safe working environment.

Employers have to do the following:

- maintain safe conditions of working with safe............(7);
- provide appropriate equipment and............(8) for the job;
- ensure that staff are............(9) in all aspects of their role;
- provide a written............(10) about health and safety in the workplace.

Equally employees need to do the following:

- co-operate with the employer and take............(11) for their own safety and that of others;
- attend training;
- ensure............(12) and documents are kept with respect to health and safety.

As required by the Act an employer has to have an ....(13) approach to these specific requirements and this requires a............(14) of the environment to be carried out. All activities within the setting must be scrutinised and potential and actual risks ....(15) and............(16). With respect to ....(17) this is a vital part of your work and as such you are likely to be trained to follow special procedures in order to ....(18) the risk to individuals in your care.

- equipment
- 'umbrella'
- records
- employer
- responsibility
- policy
- safe
- risk assessment
- infection control
- identified
- legislation
- statutory
- organised
- clothing
- employee
- trained
- minimised
- reduce

HEALTH AND SAFETY LAW

We need to understand that most of the legislation about health and safety in the workplace is based upon risk assessment and within these laws a number of requirements are laid down for work settings. These requirements are as follows.

Written policy

In an organisation where there are more than five people employed there is a requirement that a written safety policy is available to the staff. The National Minimum Standards for Care number 11.2 requires that:

> The agency delivering the care has a comprehensive health and safety policy and written procedures for health and safety management defining:
> - individual and organisational responsibilities for health and safety;
> - responsibilities and arrangements of risk assessment under the requirements of the Health and Safety at Work Regulations 1999 (management regulation).

Standard 11.2 requires that:

> The registered person appoints one or more competent persons to assist the agency in complying with their health and safety duties and responsibilities including:
> - identifying hazards and risk;
> - preparing health and safety policy statements;
> - introducing risk control measures;
> - providing adequate training and refresher training.

Within that policy the employer must show their commitment to ensuring the safety of all employees, patients/clients and others who may visit the premises by preparing a statement of intent. There should also be an implementation plan available to show how they intend to carry out that promise.

Health and safety poster or leaflet

The official Health and Safety Law poster should be displayed in all work settings (see Figure 1). On this poster there is sometimes a space in which to write the names of relevant staff who are designated either as safety officers or as first-aiders for the specific work area. Failing this, employers need to ensure that all staff are given a leaflet containing the details of the health and safety laws.

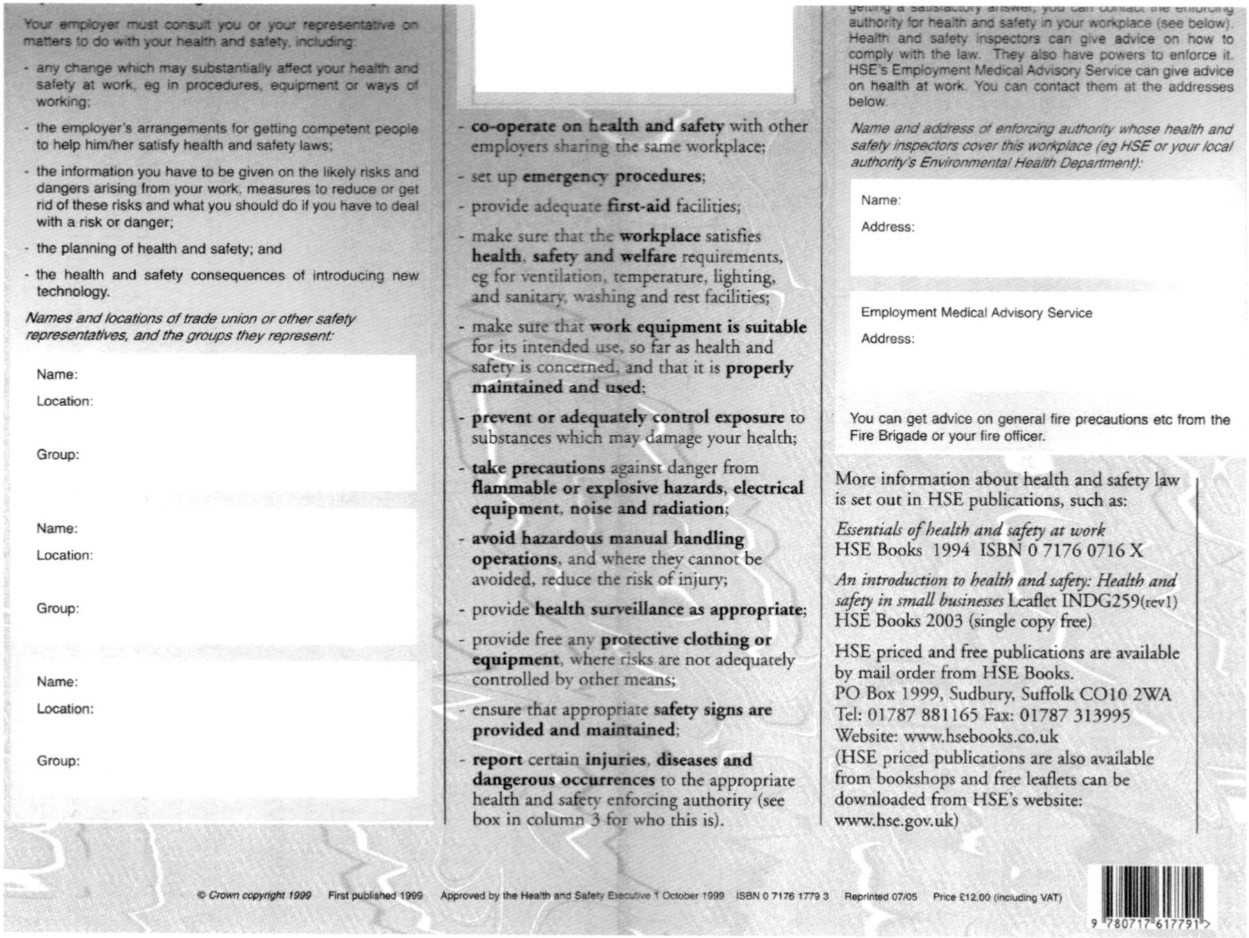

Your employer must consult you or your representative on matters to do with your health and safety, including:

- any change which may substantially affect your health and safety at work, eg in procedures, equipment or ways of working;
- the employer's arrangements for getting competent people to help him/her satisfy health and safety laws;
- the information you have to be given on the likely risks and dangers arising from your work, measures to reduce or get rid of these risks and what you should do if you have to deal with a risk or danger;
- the planning of health and safety; and
- the health and safety consequences of introducing new technology.

Names and locations of trade union or other safety representatives, and the groups they represent:

Name:
Location:
Group:

Name:
Location:
Group:

Name:
Location:
Group:

- **co-operate on health and safety** with other employers sharing the same workplace;
- set up **emergency procedures**;
- provide adequate **first-aid** facilities;
- make sure that the **workplace** satisfies **health, safety and welfare** requirements, eg for ventilation, temperature, lighting, and sanitary, washing and rest facilities;
- make sure that **work equipment is suitable** for its intended use, so far as health and safety is concerned, and that it is **properly maintained and used**;
- **prevent or adequately control exposure** to substances which may damage your health;
- **take precautions** against danger from **flammable or explosive hazards, electrical equipment, noise and radiation**;
- **avoid hazardous manual handling operations**, and where they cannot be avoided, reduce the risk of injury;
- provide **health surveillance as appropriate**;
- provide free any **protective clothing or equipment**, where risks are not adequately controlled by other means;
- ensure that appropriate **safety signs are provided and maintained**;
- **report** certain **injuries, diseases and dangerous occurrences** to the appropriate health and safety enforcing authority (see box in column 3 for who this is).

getting a satisfactory answer, you can contact the enforcing authority for health and safety in your workplace (see below). Health and safety inspectors can give advice on how to comply with the law. They also have powers to enforce it. HSE's Employment Medical Advisory Service can give advice on health at work. You can contact them at the addresses below.

Name and address of enforcing authority whose health and safety inspectors cover this workplace (eg HSE or your local authority's Environmental Health Department):

Name:
Address:

Employment Medical Advisory Service
Address:

You can get advice on general fire precautions etc from the Fire Brigade or your fire officer.

More information about health and safety law is set out in HSE publications, such as:

Essentials of health and safety at work
HSE Books 1994 ISBN 0 7176 0716 X

An introduction to health and safety: Health and safety in small businesses Leaflet INDG259(rev1)
HSE Books 2003 (single copy free)

HSE priced and free publications are available by mail order from HSE Books.
PO Box 1999, Sudbury, Suffolk CO10 2WA
Tel: 01787 881165 Fax: 01787 313995
Website: www.hsebooks.co.uk
(HSE priced publications are also available from bookshops and free leaflets can be downloaded from HSE's website: www.hse.gov.uk)

© Crown copyright 1999 First published 1999 Approved by the Health and Safety Executive 1 October 1999 ISBN 0 7176 1779 3 Reprinted 07/05 Price £12.00 (including VAT)

Figure 1 The official Health and Safety Law poster

Consultation with employees

During your induction period you will have undertaken many tasks to ensure you have knowledge about the various policies and procedures in the work setting. At this time the consultation about health and safety arrangements and how they are implemented should also have taken place.

Notification and recording of accidents

Under the Reporting of Injuries, Diseases and Dangerous Occurrences Regulations (RIDDOR) 1995 an employer is duty bound to alert the Health and Safety Executive and report any accidents that are fatal, serious or result in a person being unable to return to work for more than three days. Records must also be kept of violent incidents, work-related diseases and any injury or dangerous occurrences. Such records can be computer-based or file copies and must be housed in a safe and secure environment.

First-aid arrangements

Even though you are working in a health care environment there still needs to be a written policy and suitable arrangements for first aid. In an emergency a first-aid box must be available and a person designated to deal with the first-aid incident must also be identified. There should be a notice informing staff of the identity of the person appointed as the first-aider.

The Health and Safety Executive (HSE) is legally obliged to visit any health care premise either by prior notification or unannounced. They do this in order to check that the employer is complying with the law to safeguard their employees. It is therefore essential to clarify who is responsible for the drawing up of guidelines and policies. The following clarifies the situation:

- Premises owned by the Health Authority must refer to the contract with regard to the responsibilities for health and safety.
- Premises owned by a private owner must comply with the legislation and put into place all of the above procedures personally. They can, of course, seek help from the HSE and the Environmental Department of the local authority for guidance.

If temporary premises are used then the user must contact the owner and check that they are covered by public liability insurance.

RISK ASSESSMENT

There are a number of actual and potential risks in the workplace and whether you are moving a client or dealing with a case of MRSA your employer has a legal responsibility to carry out the appropriate risk assessments and put into place measures to minimise those risks.

In order to comply with the Safety Representatives and Safety Committee Regulations 1977 and the Health and Safety Consultations with Employees Regulations 1996 the employer needs to talk to staff in the workplace to identify the most common hazards applying to that particular area. For example, the hazards in an X-ray department are going to be vastly different to those encountered in a residential care home. However, in dealing with the outbreak of an infection or the potential passing on of infection there are certain precautions we can all take to protect ourselves. There are five steps to good risk assessment and the following will specifically apply to risk assessment of the infection control in a workplace.

Step 1: looking for hazards

There needs to be a thorough examination of the areas of practice where there might be a risk posed to staff and/or clients. In this case we are looking specifically at infection prevention and the likelihood of staff being endangered. The areas in which they may possibly be at risk of harm are in the following circumstances:

- sharps injuries;
- exposure to bodily fluids hazardous to health;
- exposure to substances and/or pathogens hazardous to health.

Step 2: who might be harmed and how?

There will of course be policies in place that specifically deal with patients and clients who are at risk of harm in the workplace, but we are concerned here with how staff might actually harm themselves in dealing with their day-to-day tasks. People coming into the workplace are also at risk and there needs to be an indication that special arrangements are made for visiting staff and public so that they are not at risk of harm.

Step 3: evaluation of the risks

There needs to be a decision made about whether the existing health and safety arrangements are adequate. If not, steps need to be taken to rectify this. For example, you may decide that your waste disposal methods are making the risk for staff greater because they have to carry infected waste further than they need to. Would changing the arrangements make it safer? If this is not possible then how can you establish safer procedures to minimise the risk?

Step 4: recording the findings

This is recommended in all places of work but is only legally required in places where there are more than five employees. Records really need to include:

- a checklist to show that a check for hazards has been made;
- that the people who might be at risk are identified;
- that the hazards and how many people might be affected are identified;
- a recommendation that existing arrangements are reasonable and that other risks are low.

Step 5: assessing the effectiveness of the precautions

After the implementation of any plan you need to check how successful and effective it has been. One of the best ways to do this is to check the written records. Following any dangerous incident staff are required to document the incident and, as outlined above, an employer is required to notify the Health and Safety Executive. If the employer finds that the accident or occurrence is one which occurs with frequency, then clearly there is a weakness in the risk assessment and this will need to be redone. There also needs to be a check that staff are in fact working to the policy in place and are aware of the risk involved.

RISKS TO YOUR OWN HEALTH IN THE WORKPLACE

Let's now look more closely at the kinds of infection prevention and control risks that you as a care worker need to be safeguarded against.

Sharps injuries and exposure to bodily fluids hazardous to health

In any setting where there is the use of injections and venepuncture the potential for injury should be noted. Staff who undertake the procedures are more at risk but the poor disposal of needles and other equipment can also prove to be a source of infection for the staff who are not directly involved in giving the injection. Staff may also be exposed to blood if they are dealing with patients who bleed as a result of injury or accident or if they are unlucky enough to be involved in violent outbursts by patients or clients. It is therefore imperative that risk assessment is undertaken to ensure that the safe disposal of needles and dressings is practised and that there are guidelines about how to minimise the risk in other incidents.

The risk to care workers in this incidence is the potential to contract hepatitis B, hepatitis C and HIV infection from the blood of patients or clients who are infected. According to the *Infection Control Guidance for Care Homes* (DoH, 2006a) the risks are as follows:

> Around one in three when a source patient is infected with hepatitis B and is 'e' antigen positive (a marker of high sensitivity), around one in 30 when the patient is infected with hepatitis C, around one in 300 when the patient is infected with HIV.

We are aware from Chapter 3 that these risks are minimised when Standard Precautions are put in place, but accidents can and do happen and, in the case of hepatitis B, staff may need to be immunised as well. However, for the other two conditions no such vaccines exist.

The risk of a needle-stick injury may be small but there should be a policy in place for the action required should such an injury occur. The following guidance should be in your policy:

• sharps should not be passed from hand to hand or person to person;
• needles should not be bent or broken;
• needles and syringes need not be dismantled prior to disposal;
• do not re-sheathe needles;
• dispose of needles into a sharps container at the point of use;
• keep the container in a safe place away from the public areas.

But what happens if, despite all the precautions above, a needle stick injury has occurred? Also, how would you deal with an accidental exposure to the blood of a client through a spillage or during a dressing or other procedure? Look at the following flow chart in Figure 2 (page 102) for guidance on what to do.

In any event where blood or bodily fluids are spilled or come into contact with persons in the workplace there is a risk that they contain high concentrations of micro-organisms and as such they must be dealt with and made safe as soon as possible.

The use of protective clothing to guard against such risks is imperative. There might also be a 'spillage kit', particularly in workplaces where this risk is high. These kits would contain a chlorine-based disinfectant and as such agents are hazardous in themselves you should always read the

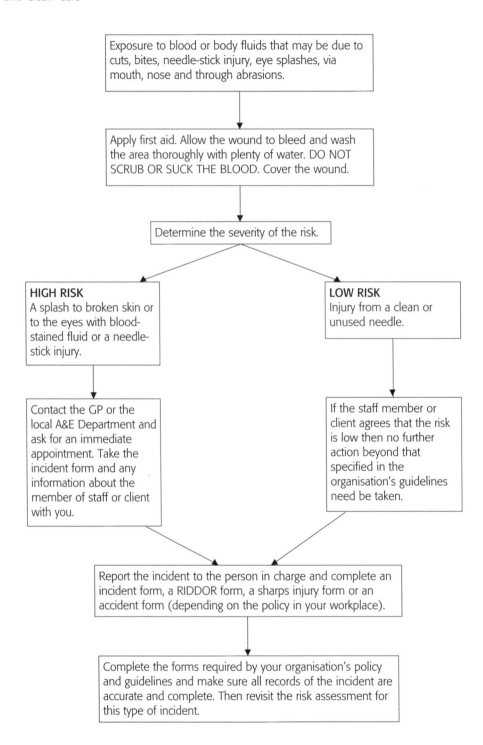

Exposure to blood or body fluids that may be due to cuts, bites, needle-stick injury, eye splashes, via mouth, nose and through abrasions.

Apply first aid. Allow the wound to bleed and wash the area thoroughly with plenty of water. DO NOT SCRUB OR SUCK THE BLOOD. Cover the wound.

Determine the severity of the risk.

HIGH RISK
A splash to broken skin or to the eyes with blood-stained fluid or a needle-stick injury.

LOW RISK
Injury from a clean or unused needle.

Contact the GP or the local A&E Department and ask for an immediate appointment. Take the incident form and any information about the member of staff or client with you.

If the staff member or client agrees that the risk is low then no further action beyond that specified in the organisation's guidelines need be taken.

Report the incident to the person in charge and complete an incident form, a RIDDOR form, a sharps injury form or an accident form (depending on the policy in your workplace).

Complete the forms required by your organisation's policy and guidelines and make sure all records of the incident are accurate and complete. Then revisit the risk assessment for this type of incident.

Figure 2 Guidance on accidental exposure to risk

manufacturer's instructions and care should be taken to avoid contact with the skin. Care should also be taken to avoid spilling disinfectants on metal surfaces as they will corrode it, or on to soft furnishings which they will bleach. Of course gloved hands must not pick up spilt needles so a scoop would also be a useful item in the kit.

The risk of infectious disease

The flow chart in Figure 2 and guidance is, of course, useful in dealing with accidental incidents as a result of which you may be in direct contact with blood, etc. but what of the infectious diseases you may come into contact with like, for example, tuberculosis? How can you take precautions against contracting such a disease?

We learned in Chapter 1 about the TB bacillus and you are encouraged to return to the relevant sections to remind yourself of the disease now. As a care worker the chances of developing such a disease are raised in the following instances:

- when in close contact with an infected person;
- when in close contact with a person who has been to a country or lived in a country where TB is common;
- when caring for homeless people, alcoholics and drug abusers who experience poor health as a result of their lifestyle.

(Unison, 2005)

The government has identified various initiatives to deal with the increasing threat of TB and key workers such as health and social care workers, residential care home and hostel workers and those in the education or public sectors are all among those who need to be informed of the risks.

To protect yourselves you need to be immunised against the disease and ensure that you work safely to reduce your risks. Your workplace risk assessment should include details of what is to be done should the need arise. You need to be tested first of all to ensure that you have the immunity needed and, if you require a vaccination, you will be offered the BCG. A chest X-ray is only necessary if you have been in close contact with a person with TB and you are considered to be at risk.

As an employer, any disease that health and social care workers may contract is covered by the COSHH regulations and any incident needs to be reported to the HSE under the RIDDOR regulations. We look in more detail at these in the next section. It is important therefore that managers are aware of the need to carry out such risk assessments if the staff in their employ are in the 'at risk' groups identified above.

Exposure to substances hazardous to health

The 2002 Control of Substances Hazardous to Health Regulations (COSHH) require employers to risk assess the substances in use in the workplace that may constitute a hazard if staff are exposed to them. The greater the risk, in terms of the severity of the outcome should exposure occur, then the greater the level of intervention to protect staff. This may require a financial commitment to provide appropriate equipment to deal with blood spills or other resources to ensure the safety of staff, or it may mean that more time is devoted to training staff to deal with such hazards. In the risk assessment the following needs to be done:

- Identify the biological hazards that are potential risks – for example, blood-borne viruses, airborne bacteria or gastric viruses.
- Assess the risks to health from exposure to these risks – for example, who is likely to suffer and how?
- Decide on the precautions to be taken – for example, Standard/Universal Precautions, hand washing, etc.
- Prevent or control the hazard – can current methods be improved or are they adequate?
- Implement a system to ensure that there is compliance with the control measures being employed.
- Ensure that employers are aware of and trained in the procedures.

(Adapted from DoH, 2006a)

RECORD KEEPING

The National Minimum Standards for Domiciliary Care number 11.4 requires that:

> All organisation records relating to Health and Safety matters are accurate and kept up to date.

Standard 4.3.1 of the common induction standards states that each care worker:

> Knows the use and purpose of each record or report the worker has to use or contribute to.

Hershey and Lawrence wrote in 1986:

> If it is not recorded then you did not do it.

These quotes emphasise the importance of the need to document and record the care given in order to provide a record that care actually took place. Of course, we could argue that merely recording what you did in no way reflects the quality of that care but we do rely on records for various reasons. Record keeping does the following:

- It provides an account of the care given.
- It assists in the making of new diagnoses and helps to define new treatment or care needed.
- It provides a record of continuous care.
- It provides a source of reference for the care workers.
- It provides a chronological account of the care from which problems can be identified.
- It provides an audit and quality assurance trail.
- It is also a legal requirement for many aspects of care.

So we need to ensure that our record keeping is:

- systematic;
- accurate;
- clear and legible.

Think about the following case study.

Case study 1

Importance of record keeping

Mrs Simms has developed a high temperature and it is not recorded. At the time it was 37.6°C. Four hours later her observations reveal a high temperature of 38.2°C and she now has a runny nose. She has been coughing and is now complaining of muscle aches. The care worker decides to put her back to bed. Four of the residents also develop coughing and sneezing and are put back to bed. The care home now has a case of influenza, which is likely to spread within the home.

Had the first record been made, Mrs Simms may well have had treatment or been isolated, which would have prevented the further spread of the condition to other clients. Her temperature was high enough to warrant further investigation. But, without the records, how was a care worker to know when her infection first became apparent and who she may have been in contact with at the time?

Records and the risk of litigation

Documentation also needs to be in place in order to protect staff and clients against the rising numbers of legal and professional litigation cases that are currently recorded. Complaints are difficult to answer if there are no adequately completed records to defend the actions of the staff. If negligence is suspected the solicitors dealing with the case will order a set of records and take statements about events from all involved. Any relevant clinical guidelines or policies will also be taken into account and the care workers' records of events will be examined. If there is any failure to carry out a procedure it will be noted and negligence may well result in further action against the care worker. Let's remind ourselves of Hershey and Lawrence's words.

If it is not recorded then you did not do it.

It is not just the recording of the care given that is important here although, as we can see from the case study above, we have no proof that we did put Mrs Simms into isolation unless we recorded that we did so. It is also the detail of the records that needs to be addressed. Should you ever be unfortunate enough to have to give evidence in a court case, you will be relieved to find that you have been diligent in the recording of the care you gave if you provide detail and measurements where necessary. Dimond (1997) highlights some of the areas of concern in care reports:

- no dates included;
- illegibility;
- use of abbreviations;
- telephone callers' names not recorded;
- no signatures;
- inaccurate times and dates;
- delay in recording care;
- allowing others to record care for you;
- inaccurate details given for clients;
- unprofessional language being used.

Therefore a checklist for the accurate recording of care will include the following:

- Have you written in a legible manner?
- Is the information in chronological order?
- Are dates and times included?
- Is there a record of how the client feels and is responding to the treatment?
- Have other relevant personnel been contacted, e.g. the infection control team?
- Has a risk assessment been carried out?
- Are there any terms used that are unprofessional or inappropriate?

• Has all transfer, discharge and admission documentation been included?

Records in infection control

It should be apparent to you now just how important records are, especially when there is an incidence of infection. Let's look back at Mrs Simms and the other residents who have just become ill.

Activity 2

To recap the situation, Mrs Simms has developed a high temperature and it has not been recorded. At the time it was 37.6°C. Four hours later her observations reveal a high temperature of 38.2°C and a runny nose. She has been coughing and is now complaining of muscle aches. The care worker decides to put her back to bed. Four of the residents also develop coughing and sneezing and are put back to bed. The care home now has a case of influenza, which is likely to spread within the home.

What records need to be made in order to ensure an action plan is put into place?

SUMMARY

The responsibility of all who work in care settings is clear. We need to provide a safe, clean and healthy environment for all our clients and patients. But equally important is the safety of care workers themselves and this chapter has set out the ways in which you can achieve this.

The need to carry out risk assessments when dealing with individuals and potentially contaminated materials is an imperative and you will have worked through an example in the first activity. By now you should be fully conversant with the way this is done in your own workplace.

Government guidance and legislation is clear. In an organisation where there are more than five people employed there is a requirement for a written safety policy to be available to the staff. The National Minimum Standards number 11.2 states that:

> a comprehensive health and safety policy and written procedures for health and safety management defining:
> • individual and organisational responsibilities for health and safety;

- responsibilities and arrangements of risk assessment under the requirements of the Health and Safety at Work Regulations 1999 (management Regulation) need to be available.

The RIDDOR guidance and the COSHH regulations require the employer to put into place safe measures with respect to reporting and assessing risks. With respect to keeping records the message is clear: 'If it is not recorded then you did not do it' (Hershey and Lawrence, 1986), emphasising the importance of the need to document and record care given in order to provide a record that care actually took place.

In the next chapter we will look more closely at the responsibility and roles in infection control.

Summary Activity

There are five steps to good risk assessment, and you are required to 'understand the need to carry out risk assessment when dealing with individuals and potentially contaminated materials.'

Identify the five stages of risk assessment for your portfolio.

Answers to the Activities

Activity 1

(1) 'umbrella'	(10) policy
(2) legislation	(11) responsibility
(3) employer	(12) records
(4) employee	(13) organised
(5) safe	(14) risk assessment
(6) statutory	(15) identified
(7) equipment	(16) minimised
(8) clothing	(17) infection control
(9) trained	(18) reduce

Activity 2

- All the clients involved should have their records up to date, including the symptoms identified and the immediate actions taken.
- If specimens are to be taken, the date and time this was carried out and when they were sent for testing should be recorded.
- The times at which they became ill needs to documented carefully.

- Other clients who have come into contact with the client should be identified and a record of their status recorded.
- Who was informed of the outbreak and at what time?
- A chronological record of events following the initial protocols being put into place needs to be clearly recorded.

Summary activity

Step 1: looking for hazards.
Step 2: who might be harmed and how?
Step 3: evaluation of the risks.
Step 4: recording the findings.
Step 5: assessing the effectiveness of the precautions.

Chapter 6

Roles, Responsibilities and Education

In this chapter you will cover the following standards:

- Skills for Care Knowledge Set on Infection Prevention and Control
  4. Roles, responsibilities and boundaries
     4.1 Understand the roles and responsibilities of personnel in relation to infection prevention and control
     4.2 Understand the roles and responsibilities of the worker with regard to following the organisation's policies and procedures
- Skills for Health Infection Prevention and Control Competencies: IPC1.

See also:
- RCN (2005a) *Good Practice in Infection Prevention and Control* – Section 10.
- NMC Essential Skills Cluster Infection Prevention and Control
  21. Patients/clients can trust a newly registered nurse to be confident in using health promotion strategies, identifying infection risks and taking effective measures to prevent and control infection in accordance with local and national policy.

INTRODUCTION

We have seen throughout the previous chapters the threat we are faced with in terms of infectious disease and the continual battle we all have against the health-care associated infections that cost our health services millions of pounds. We are well aware by now that we are all responsible for maintaining high standards of infection control in our workplaces but we need to be able to do this in a controlled and guided way if we are to succeed. Working in isolation cannot meet the needs of the twenty-first century with respect to the rising tide of newer and more virulent infections.

Legislation such as the Health and Safety at Work Act 1974, the COSHH Regulations (2002) and other professional codes of conduct (e.g. NMC) have gone a long way to ensuring that staff are accountable for their actions in maintaining a safe environment for staff, visitors, patients and clients. However, in the last two decades, the rise in HCAIs has led the government together with the Department of Health to revise current strategies and put into place certain remedies to address the issues. The Department of Health commissioned a research programme in 2000 to develop national evidence-based infection prevention and control guidelines for acute, primary and community settings. These guidelines identify a range of strategies to deal with antimicrobial resistance and reduce HCAIs in health care settings. Known as the 'EPIC initiative', these guidelines have developed broad statements of good practice and are now widely used in all care settings. Now included in all induction training for staff in health care settings the programme is rolling out to all staff, both old and new, including clinical and non-clinical workers.

ROLE OF THE INFECTION CONTROL TEAM IN HOSPITALS

Changes to the NHS in 2000 saw services being moved from the District Health Authorities to the newly formed Primary Care Trusts. Strategic health authorities replaced the old regional HAs and leadership on public health matters became firmly the role of the Directors for Public Health.

At Trust level the onus is on the Chief Executive to ensure that there are arrangements in place for the control of infection in the Trust and that programmes are implemented and monitored by specialist staff. The specialist staff comprise infection control teams (ICTs) within the Trust, made up of the infection control nurses (ICNs) and doctors (ICDs) and an infection control committee (ICC). The role of each carries the following responsibilities.

- The ICN is an expert practitioner who provides advice to staff in the hospitals and contributes to the infection control programme through teaching commitments and interpreting laboratory data to ensure the safety of the work in the Trust.
- The ICD is usually a consultant microbiologist who has a similar role to the ICN but has a key role in training doctors and medical staff.
- The ICC in each Trust comprises senior managers, the Consultant in Communicable Disease Control (CCDC), and occupational health, pharmacy and sterile supplies staff. Their remit is to endorse and make policy and to monitor the work of the infection control team and the effectiveness of the programme.
- ICTs are therefore responsible for overseeing infection prevention and control in the hospitals and PCTs around Britain.

Modern Matrons

In 2001 a new role emerged to complement the ICTs. The role of matron, which had disappeared in the 1960s, was reinstated and the modern matron was born. In order to drive up standards of care the new role was developed to 'get the basics right for patients – clean wards, good food, quality care' (DoH, 2003a).

Part of the remit of this new role was to improve the cleanliness of the wards in an effort to reduce the infections within clinical settings.

The 'Modern Matrons' report (DoH, 2003a) showed that in the period 2000–2003 £60m had been spent on improving hospital cleanliness. Figures showed the number of hospitals assessed as having 'good' standards of cleanliness increase from 23 per cent to 60 per cent. No hospitals had 'poor' cleanliness standards, which was significant when compared with the situation three years prior to the report when 35 per cent were considered poor. Ward housekeepers were in place in 45 per cent of hospitals with over 100 beds and helped improve cleaning standards by up to 30 per cent following their introduction.

One hospital, the Royal Free in London, also reported a decrease in MRSA rates following the introduction of their modern matron. This case study from the 'Modern Matrons' report showed that a matron with a hands-on role was able to support staff in implementing new initiatives such as the hand hygiene programme and brought a fresh eye to problem areas, pointing out to staff things they may have overlooked or had not previously been alerted to.

There are now more than 5000 modern matrons in post providing a strong force for improvement in care standards and ensuring cleanliness of the wards. We await further information and data from the government as to the effectiveness of this post.

THE ROLE OF INFECTION CONTROL STAFF IN THE COMMUNITY AND IN CARE HOMES

Is the picture any different in the community setting? Many workers in the social care sector work in residential or nursing homes where there are few clients. As a care home may only house a few residents an infection control team may not be in place but does this mean that infection prevention is any less of a priority than in the larger care settings?

In 2003 the National Institute for Health and Clinical Excellence published guidelines for the prevention and control of infection in the community setting to ensure that staff working in these settings were fully conversant with the measures for preventing infections associated with the use of long-term catheters, feeding systems and central venous catheters. You can view these guidelines on-line at **www.nice.org.uk**.

Also, in the social care setting, the roles and responsibilities have been identified in the Department of Health document entitled *Infection Control Guidance for Care Homes* (2006a). In Part One of this document, dealing with organisation and management, the roles are laid out as follows. Under the health and safety legislation the home owner is duty bound to ensure that there are policies in place that identify the procedures for controlling infection to ensure that all people who work in, are residents of or who enter the care home are safe at all times. This is in line with the requirements laid down by the Health Act 2006, which clearly sets out the responsibilities with respect to all aspects of infection control. The Act sets out the first responsibility of the employers as having a:

> duty to ensure, so far as is reasonably practicable, that healthcare workers are free of and are protected from exposure to communicable infections during the course of their work, and that all staff are suitably educated in the prevention and control of HCAIs.
>
> (Health Act 2006)

The registered manager must have 24-hour access to advice on infection control from qualified staff. This is where there may be a link with the Primary Care Trust, or at least with the Primary Care Group in the area. The GP has a responsibility to care for the residents in the care home and provides treatment and medications to residents when they are needed. In the case of a disease outbreak the GP must notify the Consultant in Communicable Disease Control (CCDC) who is employed by the Health Protection Agency (HPA) and has the responsibility for controlling infection in the community.

The health protection nurse (HPN) and the community infection control nurse (CICN) provide advice, education and training for the community in which they work. It is possible that the latter may work closely with the registered manager in developing policies for the care home.

You may also come across environmental health practitioners (EHPs) who, in their work for the local authority, have a remit to advise on food safety, pest control and waste disposal. The control of pollution and waste also come under their remit. Care homes are classed as food businesses and, as such, they are subject to inspections by the EPH under the Public Health (Control of Disease) Act 1984.

The Commission for Social Care Inspection (CSCI) works alongside the Health Care Commission (HCC) to ensure that all care homes are safe environments in which residents may live. Their main duties are:

- to carry out inspections in order to determine that the national minimum standards are being met, and to publish their findings;
- to register the services that meet the national minimum standards;
- to publish annual reports to parliament on national progress on social care;
- to publish star ratings for social service authorities.

So there are clearly laid down roles for the prevention of infection in the social care setting and for managing the care environment and monitoring infections.

The chain of events in the event of an infection

Activity 1

A client in your care complains of stomach cramps and develops severe diarrhoea. She has vomited once since lunchtime and has developed a raised temperature. You suspect food poisoning.

Detail the chain of events you will now put into action.

Answers to all relevant activities are given at the end of the chapter.

Your chain of events will have included members of staff in the care home as well as the GP and possibly the environmental protection officer. Whatever the outcome your initial action is most important and has to be, in the first instance, the prevention of a further outbreak in other clients. The initial isolation of the client will be the first imperative until a firm diagnosis is made and treatment can be started. The Care Standards Act 2000 clearly states that:

> The registered person shall give notice to the Commission without delay of the occurrence of the outbreak of any infectious disease which in the opinion of any registered medical practitioner attending persons in the care setting is sufficiently serious to be so notified.

Monitoring infections is an important part of your work in the care sector and the prompt diagnosis of illness will help to provide protection for staff and clients. As the GP is unlikely to be on the premises when clients get ill it is necessary for all staff to be fully trained in recognising potential outbreaks and areas for concern and that they are aware of the necessary actions to take in such an event. Symptoms in two or more patients that need to be investigated are as follows:

- cough and/or fever which may indicate an outbreak of influenza;
- diarrhoea and vomiting, which may indicate *Clostridium difficile*, noro virus or food poisoning;
- itchy skin and rash which might be due to scabies.

The Health Protection Unit will need to know of any such symptoms in two or more clients and may investigate the outbreak further. They will be there to advise the person in charge of immediate actions that need to be taken and they may also inform other agencies such as the EPO. The investigation will, in the first instance, try to establish if a problem exists and whether other clients or visitors need to be contacted to receive any extra care themselves. They will put into place measures to try to contain the outbreak where possible and limit its spread.

The likelihood of the illness spreading is of crucial importance in such a closed setting as a residential care home or a nursing home where an illness can rapidly take hold and pass to other clients. It is therefore essential that isolation of the client takes place. In most homes this is no longer a difficult task as the client can be asked to stay in their room until they are no longer infectious. However, certain resources must be put in place. There needs to be an en suite bathroom facility available to ensure that any contaminated waste product can be contained in the room and the toilet is for the sole use of the infected resident. Also hand washing facilities and waste disposal for infected linen must be available in the room. There may also be a need to employ more staff during such an outbreak since the resident may require more help than usual.

Activity 2

Access your Infection Control Policy. Does it contain the following information?

- Are biological hazards such as the risk of viral or bacterial infection identified? That is, is there a recommendation that immunisation is required for some of the infectious conditions for both staff and clients?
- Is there an identification of any substances that may cause a potential risk to staff or clients?
- Is there a list of what the standard precautions are with respect to the control of infection?
- Is there a training standard identified for staff to be informed of their role in infection control?

If your policy does not contain the above what will you do?

Hopefully you will respond to any gaps in your policy and procedures by informing the manager and identifying the means by which the gaps can be filled.

IMMUNISATION

In the last activity you were asked to make reference to your policy and there was a mention of biological hazards. This type of hazard may be prevented by vaccinations and it is a responsibility of the employer to ensure that staff and clients are all offered vaccinations if they are available and the disease is a risk to health in that particular care setting.

You may already have had vaccinations against Hepatitis B in order to protect you from exposure to the virus from contaminated blood and body fluids. Tuberculosis is another potential risk area for care workers and you may have been asked to declare whether you have been tested for and offered the BCG vaccine.

Unfortunately, an outbreak of measles has become more likely since the advent of the controversy over the MMR vaccine. Staff need to be alert to the fact that susceptible clients may well be at risk of measles from staff who have not been immunised and, in addition, your employer may require proof that you have been immunised with the MMR vaccine.

Another area of concern is the potential risk of the outbreak of flu. Influenza, as we have seen earlier, is an acute viral respiratory infection that severely affects elderly or immuno-suppressed individuals in the care setting or in the community and 12 000 deaths per year are recorded. Immunisation is offered annually to those clients who are in long-stay residential or care homes; those aged over 65 as well as to all those who may have chronic conditions such as heart, chest, liver or kidney disease or who are insulin-dependent diabetics. If you are directly involved in patient or client care you may also be offered such a vaccine in order to reduce the likelihood of the transmission of the condition to others in your care. The vaccine itself is a highly effective one and prevents influenza in working age adults. Your employer should be fully aware of the need for your clients and the staff to have an annual injection in order to reduce this risk to vulnerable clients.

THE HEALTH PROMOTION RESPONSIBILITIES OF ALL CARE WORKERS

We can spend a great deal of time fighting infections as they arise and monitoring the incidence of illness and infection. However, health care workers need to be conversant with the ways in which health may be promoted in order to avoid infection and illness altogether. According to Kenworthy *et al.* (1992) health promotion is 'the process of helping people to increase control over and improve their health'.

So how can we achieve this? The government and the health service have been instrumental in developing strategies to enhance the health of the nation. You will undoubtedly be aware of the health strategy for England *Saving Lives: Our Healthier Nation* (DoH, 1999b). In this document are to be found action plans for tackling poor health and improving the health of everyone in England. There are four priority areas for action:

- cancer – reduction in death rates by a fifth;
- coronary heart disease – reduction in death rates by two-fifths;
- accidents – reduction in death rates by a fifth;
- mental health – reduction in suicide rates by a fifth.

It was expected that the targets set nationally would be translated into local action plans and health promotion strategies would be put into place to meet the priorities. This led to the advent of campaigns to reduce smoking, reduce unemployment, improve housing, tackle pollution and improve the benefits and welfare system. We have seen the implementation of a minimum wage system to help the poorer population while the 'Sure Start' campaign ensured that children got the best start in life. Other campaigns you may also be aware of have targeted drug abuse and alcohol consumption as well as sexual health.

As health and social care workers in various settings in both hospitals and the community our responsibility to our clients is to ensure that they are fully cognisant of the means by which they can improve their own quality of life. So how does all this translate into the area in which you work? We have discussed how we reduce the risk of transmitting infection by using practical procedures such as hand washing and following these procedures can be encouraged using posters, leaflets and signage in care environments. We can also promote vaccination against infectious diseases, explain the importance of good hygiene when visiting friends and relatives in hospital and provide advice to drug users about the importance of not sharing needles. Another means may be to introduce our clients to healthy eating regimes to improve their immune systems. All of these promotional activities and many more will help to prevent and/or reduce the incidence of infection in care settings. We can also promote safe and clean care in the workplace by encouraging our colleagues to follow procedures, by being aware of the risks and taking precautions and by making sure that our own practice is as safe and clean as possible.

In order to be effective in promoting health to our clients we also need to be fully conversant with the opportunities within our local areas for improving health. For example, in the Powys region of Wales there are over-50s swimming classes and free swimming in the holidays for the children in the area. A GP referral system for gym passes is also in operation in many areas of Shropshire. As a health professional you need to be aware of the availability of such schemes for your clients in order to improve their health and well-being.

SUMMARY

We all need to take reasonable steps to reduce the possibility of infection in our clients and ourselves. Many infectious diseases are capable of spreading rapidly through any care setting and can result in enormous costs in terms of the health care required and, indeed, in terms of lives. Clear information for staff is now abundant and this chapter has shown who should bear some of the responsibility for disseminating this information to staff and patients/clients.

As a care worker you need to ensure that you are fully conversant with your responsibility with respect to preventing infections and you need to ensure that you are continually updating your knowledge.

Having worked through all the chapters in the book you should now be in a good position to demonstrate your knowledge of many aspects of infection prevention and control. Think about all the evidence you have collected and talk to your mentor/manager about how this may be presented to demonstrate your participation in continuing professional development.

Infection control in any care setting is the responsibility of all who work or enter the setting and we as care workers need to educate others to ensure that we are all working together to reduce the deaths from infection.

Perhaps Florence Nightingale, a tireless campaigner for cleaner hospitals, should have the last word, and for 'nursing' perhaps we can also read 'care work' to bring the terminology up to date:

> True nursing ignores infection, except to prevent it. Cleanliness and fresh air from open windows, with unremitting attention to the patient, are the only defence a true nurse either asks or needs. Wise and humane management of the patient is the best safeguard against infection.
>
> (Nightingale, 1860)

Patient or client care that is delivered with a high level of knowledge and regard to the standard precautions required for the prevention of infection is the only way we can be assured of safe, clean care and infection prevention.

Answers to Activities

Activity 1

The client needs to be isolated immediately so she must be returned to her room and special precautions put into place straightaway. Visitors to the home should be restricted and, if they are present, they should avoid close contact with the patient. Other people living in the same home should also limit contact with the patient. Any soiled linen must be dealt with as per the protocols in place and bagged and disposed of as infected waste. You need to alert the person in charge of the change in the client's condition who will then inform other staff of the potential infection risk. The person in charge will ring the GP who will visit to diagnose and treat the client. The GP will then notify the local authority's officer such as the CCDC.

If the infection is due to food then a sample of the suspected food will need to be kept and the environmental protection officer will be informed and lead an investigation.

Glossary

aerobe   a micro-organism that requires oxygen to survive/reproduce.

amino acids   the building blocks of proteins.

anaerobe   a micro-organism that does not require oxygen to survive/reproduce.

Anopheles   a genus of mosquito – the females can transmit the *Plasmodium* parasite that causes malaria.

antigens   proteins on the cell surface that trigger an immune response.

bacteriocidal   capable of killing bacteria.

bacteriostatic   inhibit the growth or multiplication of bacteria.

bacterium   a single-celled prokaryotic organism.

binomial   a two-term scientific name for a living organism, e.g. *Homo sapiens*.

broad spectrum antibiotics   affecting a wide variety of bacterial species.

Candida albicans   the single-celled fungus that causes thrush.

cerumen   waxy substance most commonly found in the ear canal.

chlamydia   a pathogenic bacterium.

clinical governance   an umbrella term describing the quality functions and effective use of risk management and evidence-based practice in clinical work.

Clostridium tetanii   the anaerobic bacteria that causes tetanus (lockjaw).

colonisation   when a population of bacteria may survive on or in a person but not cause disease.

commensal   an organism that lives in association with other organisms.

communicable   a disease that can be transmitted from one person to another.

complement   a set of proteins that bind to pathogens/antigens and promote phagocytosis.

cystic fibrosis   an inherited disease that results in the formation of very thick sticky mucous, affecting the lungs, pancreas and reproductive organs.

cytology   the study of cells.

cytoplasm   the contents of a cell excluding its organelles.

cytotoxic   toxic to cells.

Deep Clean Initiative measure introduced by the government in 2008 to tackle health care associated infections and ensure patient safety and confidence by introducing extensive cleaning in clinical areas.

endospores – see *spores*.

enzymes a group of proteins that catalyse reactions in living organisms.

ESBLs extended-spectrum β lactamases – a group of enzymes produced by some pathogens that enable them to breakdown antibiotics.

Escherichia coli a bacterium that can be both commensal and pathogenic depending on the strain.

eukaryotes cells/organisms with a nucleus.

fertilisation the fusing of a sperm with an ovum.

flagella a cell organelle that enables the cell to move.

genes sections of DNA that code for a particular protein.

Golgi body/apparatus a eukaryotic cell organelle that prepares protein for secretion.

Gram negative bacteria that stain pink with Gram stain.

Gram positive bacteria that stain purple with Gram stain.

Gram staining a technique used to distinguish between Gram positive and Gram negative bacteria.

immunity the body's ability to fight infection.

inherited a characteristic or disease that is received from parents via genes.

insulin a hormone produced by the pancreas that reduces blood sugar.

Klebsiella a genus of bacteria.

lipids a group of biochemicals, e.g. fats, oils and waxes.

lysosome a eukaryotic cell organelle that contains digestive enzymes.

mesosome a folding in the cell membrane of bacteria that is thought to be the site of respiration.

microbes living organisms too small to be seen with the naked eye.

micrometre a thousandth of a millimetre.

micro-organisms – see *microbes*.

microvilli folds in the surface membrane of animal cells that increase the surface area for absorption.

multicellular made of many cells.

Mycobacterium bovis a bacterium that causes TB in cattle.

narrow spectrum antibiotics affecting only a few bacterial species.

nucleus a eukaryotic cell organelle that contains chromosomes.

parasites multicellular organisms that live on or in a host and cause it harm.

pathogens   disease-causing micro-organisms.

Pediculus capitis   head lice.

phagocyte   white blood cell that engulfs and destroys pathogens.

plasmid   a small loop of DNA that can be transferred between bacteria.

Plasmodium   – see *Anopheles*.

prokaryotes   single-celled organisms without a nucleus.

proteins   a diverse group of molecules found in all living organisms with a range of functions.

ribosome   a very small cell organelle that makes protein in both eukaryotes and prokaryotes.

rough endoplasmic reticulum   a system of membranes in eukaryotic cells that is covered with ribosomes, the site of protein synthesis.

Salmonella typhi   the pathogen that causes typhoid fever.

smooth endoplasmic reticulum   a system of membranes in eukaryotic cells that is not covered with ribosomes; the site of steroid and lipid synthesis.

sperm   the male gamete.

spores   reproductive structures produced by bacteria, lower plants and fungi.

Standard Universal Precautions   set of principles designed to prevent the transmission of HIV, hepatitis B and other blood-borne pathogens.

Streptococcus pneumoniae   the pathogen that causes pneumonia.

syphilis   a sexually transmitted disease.

typhoid fever   a disease caused by *Salmonella typhi* transmitted by the oral/faecal route.

unicellular   made up of one cell.

vector   an organism that transmits a pathogen from host to host, for example the female *Anopheles* mosquito is a vector for the *Plasmodium* parasite that causes malaria.

References

Audit Commission (1997) *Getting Sorted: The Safe and Economical Management of Hospital Waste.* Abingdon: Audit Commission Publications

Ayliffe, G.A.J. (1993) *Chemical Disinfection in Hospitals.* London: Public Health Laboratory Service

Ayliffe, G.A.J., Babb, J.R. and Qouraishi, A.H. (1978) 'A test for "hygienic" hand disinfection'. *Journal of Clinical Pathology,* 31: 923–8

Babb, J.R., Davies, J.G. and Ayliffe, G.A.J. (1983) 'Contamination of protective clothing and nurses' uniforms in an isolation ward'. *Journal of Hospital Infection,* 4: 49–57

Centers for Disease Control (1987) 'Recommendations for prevention of HIV transmission in health-care settings'. *Morbidity and Mortality Weekly Report,* 36 (suppl. no. 2): 3–18

Centers for Disease Control (1988) 'Agent summary statement for human immunodeficiency virus and report on laboratory-acquired infection with human immunodeficiency virus'. *Morbidity and Mortality Weekly Report,* 37 (suppl. no. 14): 1–22

Department of Health (1996) *Methicillin Resistant* Staphylococcus aureus *in Community Settings.* London: DoH

Department of Health (1998) *A First Class Service: Quality in the New NHS.* London: DoH

Department of Health (1999a) *Resistance to Antibiotics and Other Antimicrobial Agents: Action for the NHS Following the Government's Response to the House of Lords Science and Technology Committee report 'Resistance to Antibiotics and Other Antimicrobial Agents'.* London: DoH

Department of Health (1999b) *Saving Lives: Our Healthier Nation.* London: DoH

Department of Health (2000a) *Domiciliary Care – National Minimum Standards.* London: HMSO

Department of Health (2000b) *The Management and Control of Hospital Acquired Infection in Acute NHS Trusts in England,* HC 230 Session 1999–00. London: DoH

Department of Health (2000c) *The Management and Control of Hospital Infection: Action for the NHS for the Management and Control of Infection in Hospitals in England,* Health Service Circular HSC (2000) 2. London: DoH

Department of Health (2002) *Getting Ahead of the Curve: A Strategy for Combating Infectious Diseases (Including Other Aspects of Health Protections): A Report by the Chief Medical Officer.* London: DoH

Department of Health (2003a) *Modern Matrons – Improving the Patient Experience.* London: DoH.

Department of Health (2003b) *Surveillance of Health Care Associated Infections,* letter from the Chief Medical Officer: PLCMO 2003. London: DoH

Department of Health (2003c) *Winning Ways: Working Together to Reduce Healthcare Associated Infection in England.* London: DoH. Available on-line at: **www.dh.gov.uk/en/Publicationsandstatistics/Publications/PublicationsPolicy**

AndGuidance/Browsable/DH_4095070 (accessed 6 August 2008)

Department of Health (2004a) *Mandatory C. difficile Surveillance Scheme – Reports by Category October 2003 – September 2004.* London: DoH.

Department of Health (2004b) *Mandatory GRE Bacteraemia Surveillance Scheme – GRE Reports by Category October 2003 – September 2004.* London: DoH

Department of Health (2004c) *Mandatory MRSA Surveillance Scheme – Reports by Category October 2003 – September 2004.* London: DoH

Department of Health (2004d) *Stopping Tuberculosis in England.* London: DoH

Department of Health (2004e) *Towards Cleaner Hospitals and Lower Rates of Infection. A Summary of Action.* London: DoH

Department of Health (2005) *Saving Lives: A Delivery Programme to Reduce Health Care-Associated Infection Including MRSA.* London: DoH

Department of Health (2006a) *Infection Control Guidance for Care Homes.* London: DoH

Department of Health (2006b) *Safe Management of Healthcare Waste,* Health Technical Memorandum 07-01. London: DoH

Department of Health (2006c) *The Health Act 2006 – Code of Practice for the Prevention and Control of Healthcare Associated Infections.* London: DoH

Department of Health (2006d) *Essential Steps to Safe, Clean Care: Reducing Healthcare-associated Infections.* London: DoH

Department of Health (2007a) *A Simple Guide to* Clostridium difficile. London: HMSO

Department of Health (2007b) *Essential Steps Towards Cleaner Hospitals.* London: DoH

Dimond, B. (1997) *Legal Aspects of Care in the Community.* Basingstoke: Macmillan

Dowsett, E.G. and Wilson, P.A. (1981) 'An outbreak of *Streptococcus pyogenes* in a maternity unit'. *CDR*, 81(17): 3

Greaves, A. (1985) 'We'll just freshen you up, dear'. *Nursing Times*, 6 March (suppl.): 3–8

Health and Safety Executive (2002) *Control of Substances Hazardous to Health Regulations.* London: HSE

Health and Safety Executive (2003) *Essential Information for Providers of Residential Accommodation.* Suffolk: HSE

Health Protection Agency (2005a) *MRSA Surveillance System: Results.* DoH: London

Health Protection Agency (2005b) *Pandemic Flu: UK Influenza Pandemic Contingency Plan.* London: TSO

Health Protection Agency (n.d.) *Tuberculosis.* On-line at: **www.hpa. org.uk/infections/topics_az/tb/data_menu.htm** (accessed 16 September 2008)

Health Services Advisory Committee (1999) *Safe Disposal of Clinical Waste.* London: HMSO

Hershey, N. and Lawrence, R. (1986) 'The influence of charting upon liability determination'. *Journal of Nursing Administration*, 35/37, March/April

House of Lords Science and Technology Committee (1998) Resistance to Antibiotics and Other Antimicrobial Agents. London: TSO **www.parliament.the-stationery-office.co.uk/pa/ld199798/ldsctech081 vii/std701.htm**

Indge, W. (2003) *Complete A–Z Biology Handbook.* London: Hodder & Stoughton

Ison, E. (1998) *Analysis of Acute and Community Hospital Clinical Waste.* National Household Hazardous Waste Forum Autumn Meeting, November

Jones, K. (1994) 'Waterborne diseases'. *New Scientist*, 9 July

Kenworthy, N., Snowley, G. and Gilling, C. (1992) *Common Foundation Studies in Nursing.* London: Churchill Livingstone.

McGinley, K.L., Larson, E.L. and Leyden, J.J. (1988) 'Composition and density of microflora in the subungual space of the hand'. *Journal of Clinical Microbiology*, 26: 950–3

Medical Devices Agency (1996) *Parts 1 and 2 – Sterilisation, Disinfection and Cleaning of Medical Equipment – Guidance on Decontamination from the Microbiology Advisory Committee to Department of Health Medical Devices Agency.* London: TSO

Moolenaar, R.L., Crutcher, J.M., San Joaquin, V.H., Sewell, L.V., Hutwagner, L.C., Carson, L.A., Robison, D.A., Smithee, L.M.K. and Jarvis, W.R. (2000) 'A prolonged outbreak of *Psuedomonas aeruginosa* in a neonatal intensive care unit: did staff fingernails play a role in disease transmission?' *Journal of Infection Control and Hospital Epidemiology*, 21: 80–5

National Institute for Clinical Excellence (2003) *Infection Control: Prevention of Healthcare-Associated Infection in Primary and Community Care.* London: NICE

National Statistics Office (n.d.) *MRSA.* **www.statistics.gov.uk/CCI/nugget.asp? ID=1067** (accessed 1 December 2007)

Nightingale, F. (1860) *Notes on Nursing.* New York: Appleton

Nikiforuk, A. (1991) *The Fourth Horseman.* London: Fourth Estate

Pellow, C.M., Pratt, R.J., Harper, P., Loveday, H.P., Robinson, N., Jones, S., MacRae, E.D. and the Guideline Development Group for NICE (2003) *Prevention of Health Care Associated Infections in Primary and Community Care.* London: NICE

Perry, C., Marshall, I.R. and Jones, I.E. (2001) 'Bacterial contamination of uniforms'. *Journal of Hospital Infection*, 48: 238–41

Plowman, R., Graves, N., Griffin, M., Roberts, J.A., Swan, A.V., Cookson, B. and Taylor, L. (1999) *The Socio-Economic Burden of Hospital Acquired Infections.* London: Public Health Laboratory Service

Porter, R. (1997) *The Greatest Benefit to Mankind: A Medical History from Antiquity to the Present.* London: HarperCollins

Postgate, J. (1992) *Microbes and Man.* Cambridge: Cambridge University Press

Pratt, R.J., Pellowe, C., Loveday, H.P., Robinson, N., Smith, G.W., Barrett, S., Davey, P., Harper, P., Loveday, C., McDougall, C., Mulhall, A., Privett, S., Smales, C., Taylor, L., Weller, B. and Wilcox, M. (2001) 'The EPIC Project: developing national evidence-based guidelines for preventing health care associated infections. Phase 1: guidelines for preventing hospital acquired infections'. *Journal of Hospital Infection*, 47 (suppl.): S3–S82

Royal College of Nursing (2005a) *Good Practice in Infection Prevention and Control.* London: RCN

Royal College of Nursing (2005b) *Guidance on Uniform and Clothing Worn in the Delivery of Patient Care.* London: RCN

Smith, H. (1995) 'How bacteria cause disease'. *Biological Sciences Review*, 7(3): 2

Taylor, L. (1978) 'An evaluation of handwashing techniques'. *Nursing Times*, 74: 108–10

UK Clostridium Difficile Support (n.d.) **www.cdiff-support.co.uk**. (accessed 30 July 2008)

Unison (2005) *Tuberculosis*, Health and Safety Information Sheet. Available online: **www.unison.org.uk** (accessed 25 August 2008).

Volk, W.A., Benjamin, D.C., Kadner, R.J. and Parsons, J.T. (1991) *Essentials of Medical Microbiology.* Philadelphia: J. P. Lippincott

World Health Organization (2006a) *Building on and Enhancing DOTS to Meet the TB-Related Millenium Developmental Goals.* Geneva: WHO

World Health Organization (2006b) *Global Tuberculosis Control: Surveillance, Planning and Financing*, WHO Report WHO/HTM/TB.2006.362. Geneva: WHO.

Index

Added to a page number 'f' denotes a figure and 't' denotes a table.